D1276007

Date: 6/16/17

617.412 BUL
Bull, Kate,
Open hearts :stories of the
surgery that changes children's

Open Hearts

Open Hearts

**Stories of the Surgery that
Changes Children's Lives**

KATE BULL

First published 2016 by
Elliott and Thompson Limited
27 John Street
London WC1N 2BX
www.eandtbooks.com

ISBN: 978-1-78396-227-3

Poem on p. 274, 'Taking You There' by Rebecca Goss, from *Her Birth*, Carcanet Press
Ltd, 2013. Reprinted with permission.

Plate section: Page 1: Museum Arnhem; photograph by Peter Cox; Page 2: Photo by
James Burke/Time & Life Pictures/Getty Images; Page 3, top: Photo by Al Fenn/
The LIFE Picture Collection/Getty Images; Page 3, bottom: Hospital Archives,
The Hospital for Sick Children, Toronto, with permission; Page 4, top: Medical
Photography Department, Great Ormond Street Hospital, with permission; Page 4,
bottom: Family photo, with permission; photograph by Pat Butler; Page 5: Family
photo, with permission; photograph by Ken Schmohe; Page 6: Michael Toon personal
collection, with permission; Page 7: Family photo, with permission; Page 8: 'Scarred
for Life' is a Somerville Foundation initiative; photograph by Kirsty Anderson.

Diagrams on pp. 294–296 by Jon Wainwright.

9 8 7 6 5 4 3 2 1

A catalogue record for this book is available from the British Library.

Typesetting: Marie Doherty
Printed in the UK by TJ International Ltd

*Thanks to
Jane Somerville.
We owe you.*

CONTENTS

Introduction   1

1 Beginnings   7
2 Minnesota, Tuesday 31 August 1954   11
3 When nothing is done   29
4 Birth was almost the death of him   45
5 'Those children are my crossword puzzles'   57
6 When did you last see a blue baby?   79
7 Going into hospital   95
8 Magic sleep   115
9 Cold hearts   129
10 'It's a very detailed and complex operation . . .'   147
11 This won't hurt a bit: recovery   159
12 Finding a new normal: after surgery   179
13 Dirty washing   187
14 Flying solo   197
15 Grown up and trying to do normal things   217
16 Having a baby – what's the big deal?   231
17 Rhythm problems and other woes: the rise of the expert
   patient   241
18 'Death alone is certain, the time of death is uncertain'   257
19 What's new? (Besides innovation)   275

   Appendix   293
   Acknowledgements   297
   References   299
   Index   305

INTRODUCTION

$\mathfrak{I}$ had a 1950s and 1960s childhood. Every summer we went to the same caravan park in the same sand dunes in Donegal and our first ritual on arrival was to take our pocket money to the shack-shop to buy a bar of Cadbury's Mint Crisp, not sold in Belfast. The shop-family had two daughters, both older than I was, who never strayed from the step outside. Even the six-year-old me could see that they were 'different' and, knowing what I do now, I realize that both had Down's syndrome. The sisters had the sameness of twins, but it was not their almond-shaped eyes or the way they held their tongues or their incurious manner that was so striking. They were definitely the wrong colour. Their lips were a dark, dark purple, their eyes were cerise and their complexions a weird blue. Children are told not to stare, but I promise that, even as an adult, you would have taken a second look. I referred my 'why' to my parents. Both doctors, they gave me my very first lesson about hearts and what you can deduce from appearances; for some years I became a proper little Sherlock Holmes. There came a year when only one girl was on the step.

Nowadays, if you ask people younger than a certain age when they last saw a 'blue baby', they often look a bit blank. With the march of progress, the phrase 'blue baby' has disappeared from the vernacular, along with children blue enough to stop us in the street. Before surgery became available, children born with badly organized hearts lived out the 'natural history' of whatever defect they were born with, their bodies succumbing to the lethargy of living without an efficient circulation. Some would survive days, others to school age; very few became young adults who we might see out and about. Before the early 1960s, newborn babies were not rushed to specialist hospitals as they are today. The few surgeons of the time with any know-how would not have operated on them anyway; surgery was reserved for older and physically bigger children – and hardly any babies with critical heart disease would live to grow to their target size for having an operation.

The very first operation on a blue baby took place in the Johns Hopkins Hospital in Baltimore in late 1944. The surgeon was Alfred Blalock, who went on to visit London to perform the first operation in Europe in 1947. The variety of congenital heart disease is prodigious but his operation benefited a group of children who were blue because their lung-blood supply was restricted by some blockage inside their hearts. In the 1940s, the heart itself was still 'off limits' to surgeons, but Blalock's operation redirected blood heading to the child's left arm and diverted it into their lung arteries. These operations were palliative – the problems inside their hearts remained – but their effects were dramatic; the extra oxygen that the shunt afforded to the children's bodies was life-changing. By the early 1950s, American surgeons were beginning to operate inside children's hearts – accounts of their staggeringly low-tech equipment (ice baths, circuits mingling a parent's blood with their child's) will turn up in this book. These operations yielded the earliest survivors of 'open-heart surgery', and some recount their sides of the stories for us.

By the 1960s, confidence, competence and the availability of expertise led to an increase in the numbers arriving at hospitals in the hope of treatment, though the death rate for babies before, during and after surgery was still prohibitively high. The most straightforward defects were necessarily the first to be tackled, but over the next two decades major technological improvements – in diagnosis, anaesthesia and intensive care as well as surgery – meant that by the late 1980s the list of congenital heart problems that could not be alleviated at all had shrunk to almost nothing.

At the beginning, children had to be quite disabled by their hearts before surgeons could justify the risk of operating, so many of the early survivors remember their lives before, during and after their surgery. Some have offered to talk to a curious veteran from the other side of the doctor-patient relationship – for instance offering their perspective on the atmosphere of children's wards. Some had been dragged from their parents on admission to hospital, nurses had sometimes been unsympathetic, stays had been long and parental visiting might only be allowed once a week. In such an environment, children look out for the good people, and there are also accounts of heart-stopping acts of kindness. The climate of children's wards has changed but, related to the advances described in this book, most contemporary children born with heart problems have had their 'main' operation by the time they go to school (making most of them pink or nearly pink) and unlike their predecessors, most have no memory of their own life-or-death crises – ordeals that parents of every era remember only too well.

For the avoidance of doubt, 'blue babies' are still out there – you simply have not noticed them. From a class photograph, I doubt you would pick out the child with only 'half a heart' who had already undergone an arduous series of operations before he was five years old – though you might spot him if you watched carefully on the sports field. Currently, in Britain alone, over 1,000 heart operations are performed every year on babies before they are even one month old. In the USA – thanks to childhood surgery – more than one million adults are now thought to be living with heart diseases that they were born with. Numerically, congenital heart disease is no longer primarily a problem of childhood – indeed, for the past twenty years, affected adults have outnumbered the children. With numbers like these, we have to wonder why we have not met one of the people this book is about. We probably have. Most patients keep their scars well hidden and many told me how 'our' many misconceptions make them cautious about who they tell.

The whole project of heart surgery on children has been a 'gift that keeps on giving' for the press, who love a triumphalist narrative of a surgeon meeting a challenge. This cliché is careless for several reasons. Firstly a child's survival through surgery depends as much on the rest of their team's competence in preoperative diagnosis, anaesthesia and post-operative intensive care; we hear how these evolved over the decades. Secondly, even now, few operations offer a 'cure'. This means that many survivors are negotiating adult life with disabilities from incomplete repairs and some are squaring up to premature death. Finally and most unfairly, the part played by trailblazing patients is completely unacknowledged.

Blalock and many of the early 'open heart' surgeons became international celebrities, yet as accounts of burgeoning numbers of novel heart operations came to appear in the medical press, the patients' identities were always redacted. But it is the patients' stories that form the backbone of this book. No less than the surgeons, they were truly pioneers, yet no acknowledgement is ever made of how crucial they were to events. Until recently, most of them had never encountered anyone else who had had similar surgery. But now – like people who research their family history – patients use the internet to get in touch with others who share their diagnosis and the oldest patients are like the elders of a scattered tribe.

Almost all of my professional experience has been at the child-hood end of congenital heart disease services, though I looked at my profession from another angle during the treatment of my own child for a queer cancer. That experience also taught me that

– when a doctor takes their eyes off their 'patients' – they are not 'patients' at all, just kids trying to get on with their lives. This was the beginning of my interest in the stories of out-of-hospital lives.

Most of the 'patients' I talked to – in person, by Skype or over the telephone – I 'met' as strangers; it has been curious to have the doctor-patient relationship out of the way. To have an hour, sometimes two, occasionally a couple of days to spend with people is not something that ever happens in a hospital out-patient clinic. As doctors, we undoubtedly bear witness to what patients go through in hospital, but listening is another matter. Questions went back and forth in both directions; I think many of them enjoyed the sessions. They have been mainly adults – most children struggle one-to-one with an inquisitive stranger. We went through their life stories in much the same way that the book is constructed: birth, diagnosis, childhood, hospitals . . . Some had become parents themselves and had only then recognized what their own families had been through. A particular privilege for me were the pensive conversations with survivors of early operations for conditions that were edgy at the time but that we now think of as routine – Fallot, VSD (conditions that are explained more fully later). These were people of my own generation and it was poignant to hear them decades later describing their pin-bright recollections of fleeting childhood incidents in family life or the school playground. Memory is fickle; we forget what we want to remember and remember what we want to forget. But in the back of my mind I was constantly wondering how today's children, born with the problems that are now on the margin of our capabilities – Hypoplastic Left Heart, complex pulmonary atresia, single ventricle – will look back on their childhoods in forty years' time.

As may become evident if you read on, I have become a fan of what has come to be called the 'Adult Congenital Heart' community. Their very existence has been framed as a triumph of human progress over nature – but this tells only the 'medical' part of the story. The early patients were pathfinders; their survival launched them into uncharted waters. Incognito in books about the history of medicine – and often living 'incognito' among us – I believe they deserve more credit. Father Patrick (who you will first meet as a four-year-old learning to walk in a 1960s hospital ward) chides me for my 'rose-tinted' admiration of the 'graduates' of our surgery. He has good judgement, but I am not going to apologize for my admiration. To them I say: 'Don't underestimate what you have done.'

1
Beginnings

Making a blue child pink is one of the great stunts of modern medicine. Cosmetic surgery can change a face or a breast, but the first 'reveal' after these operations looks worse than before the surgeon started – stitching, bruising and distortion all take time to settle. But there is a moment in every operation on a blue baby when the scale of the transformation in the child's appearance is revealed, the anaesthetist at the head of the table smiles, and an hour later the baby's parents can hardly believe their eyes. The stereotypical surgeon is much harder to impress.

The year was 1947. Even Fellows of the Royal College of Surgeons of London start glancing at their watches, shifting in their seats and looking forward to a drink after two weighty lectures. The speakers were Drs Helen Taussig and Alfred Blalock who, in 1944, had accomplished the first ever operation on a 'blue baby' at the Johns Hopkins Hospital in Baltimore. The 'blueness' of their patients was plain for all to see. Born with a defect inside their hearts that blocked the way through to their lungs, their blood was short of oxygen, their energy levels pitiful and most would die after a short and sorry life.

Between 1945 and 1947, youngsters had been arriving by the

hundreds at Blalock's hospital, blue and in wheelchairs, and the lucky ones had been trotting out pink and unaided a fortnight later. The success rate had improved and the operation standard-ized to the extent that Blalock could begin teaching it to other surgeons. His visit to Guy's Hospital in London was his first trip outside the USA. There, with the local chief Russell Brock, he had spent a week operating on eight children. Before returning to the USA, Blalock was invited to address his eminent surgical audience. Realizing that history was being made, someone had recorded a flickering cine film showing the two surgeons at work; with 1947 film, lighting and lenses, it cannot have given much more than a record of the cast-list. The lights in the auditorium were dimmed for the cine and there was some shuffling on stage. Then, as Brock remembered:

> a long searchlight beam traversed the whole length of the hall and unerringly picked out on the platform a Guy's nursing sister in her attractive blue uniform, sitting on a chair and holding a small cherub-like girl of 2½ years with a halo of blond curly hair and looking pink and well. It was a Madonna like tableau . . . no one there could possibly forget it.

Unbelievably, there was a standing ovation. Surgery for congenital heart disease, born in the USA, started in Europe that day.

Beginnings are exciting times and the legacies of Blalock and Brock are assured.* The operations that each championed are named after them and both published many medical papers. After his lecture, the Royal College of Surgeons festooned Blalock with

---

* Though as it turned out, neither man was temperamentally suited to the next challenge in congenital heart surgery: operating inside the heart itself required teamwork.

bling and braid; later, Brock became an English lord. The first Baltimore operations have even been immortalized in a Hollywood film, *Something the Lord Made* (2004) – though this was a revisionist account and the title referred not to Blalock's surgical skill but that of his African-American lab assistant.

Though we know that the very first baby to receive a Blalock shunt was called Eileen Saxon; she only survived for a few months. Nothing further is known of the little girl on the nurse's lap. As she grew, the amount of blood going through her shunt would have gradually failed to meet her body's oxygen needs and her energy levels must have declined as she became become bluer again. The radical solution of opening up her heart to deal with the problems inside it was more than a decade away in England. Again, the 'first' was to be in the USA.

2
Minnesota, Tuesday 31 August 1954

Spectators looking down through the glass ceiling above a Minneapolis operating room witnessed a drama of first-night unpredictability playing out below them. The operating table looked like a kitchen table, neatly laid with a green cloth, and with shiny steel silverware arranged at one end. Androgynous figures, hatted and masked, indistinguishable in loose-fitting gowns, stooped close together, arms sometimes entwined; the usual conventions about personal space being suspended in an operating room. Within the central tableau, a bright spotlight drew attention to the compelling spectacle of a dark-red beating heart. Choreographed activities with an insistent momentum played out in the central huddle; esoteric sub-plots were discernible outside the spotlight. There were pauses with everyone standing stock-still as their attention converged. There was blood. All the drama somehow distracted from what was concealed under the green cloth.

Surgeons have often been painted as the main protagonists in the war against congenital heart disease. Portrayed as generals, some have been tacticians, others technicians, some prudent, others reckless. Some have rightly been decorated for their roles in the campaign, a few have become celebrities. But not one of these surgeons ever faced the prospect of dying on the battlefield. This book tells the story of the people underneath the green drapes, and in this particular operating theatre there were two.

★　★　★

In 1944, Mickey Shaw's life had an inauspicious start. The nurses whose job it was to wrap up babies for their homeward journeys in a Minnesota February gave Mickey's mother the wrong baby. Unpacking her bundle in her bedroom at home, there ensued one of those set-piece episodes that only seem funny in retrospect – a drive at breakneck speed, red-faced staff, two frantic mothers.

Young Mickey Shaw never really thrived; a puny baby, late to walk. He was the second of four sons but his little brother soon outgrew him. He walked exasperatingly slowly – half a block would leave him breathless. He would stop, squat and hug his knees to his chest, looking blue enough to alarm passers-by. By the time he was going to school, the whole town must have been aware of him being towed along by a reluctant brother on a wagon that the family used for groceries. 'Heart problem' was an easy call for the school doctor, who suggested that his mother take him to see a specialist in Minneapolis-St Paul which, although only sixty miles to the east, was a whole world away; locals called the twin cities 'Sodom and Gomorrah'.

There, in 1950, Mickey had some tests, including a cardiac catheterization. The doctors opened a vein in the crook of his elbow and – watching on cine X-ray – ran a plastic tube towards and through his heart, taking blood samples on the way to track how the red and blue blood was streaming. By the end of a week, they had a name for Mickey's condition. His blue colour was due to a shortage of oxygen in his blood and that in turn explained his lack of stamina. It is unlikely that the specialist conveyed much of the anatomy of Tetralogy of Fallot* to Mickey's mother, but the implications were explicit. 'Sadly' he had a heart problem; 'yes' the problems were right inside his heart; 'no' there was nothing they could do and 'yes' he would die before he was sixteen. Mickey Shaw's name, address and diagnosis was put on a card and added to a growing file of children with inoperable heart defects.

Mickey's mother, Helen, was a more than decent woman: a good Catholic whose husband had abandoned her with no maintenance soon after the fourth boy was born. Rather than accept welfare, she did cleaning jobs on Saturday and Sunday afternoons and on weekdays worked in an industrial freezing unit, standing in an inch of water eviscerating turkeys. Her boys were lively but polite and well groomed. The family dressed neatly for Mass on Sundays and said grace before meals. Respecting her dignity, shopkeepers may have put a few dented cans her way and the nuns at school very probably looked out for Mickey. These were the days when pupils were taught how to 'duck and cover' in the event of nuclear war; a time of bikes and milkshakes and freeze-dried jeans and the Lone Ranger on the radio.

When the press began to publish news of heart operations on children in Baltimore, Helen wrote a pleading letter to the director of the hospital. In principle a Blalock shunt would have helped Mickey, but in practice, with no family money and no local expertise, there was no operation on offer. She became despondent – three boys boisterous and one gradually deteriorating. It was painful on some evenings for her loyal sons, each trying to help with paper rounds and lawn-mowing jobs, to overhear their uncomplaining mother crying in her room.

Then in March 1954 another letter arrived, inviting them back to Minneapolis, this time to meet a surgeon who offered

---

* Tetralogy of Fallot a.k.a Fallot's Tetralogy, 'Fallot' or 'Tetralogy' or 'Tet'.

some hope. He was prepared to try a completely new approach –
to operate inside Mickey's heart. In her straitened circumstances,
money was the first problem that panicked Helen, but the surgeon
promised that the research fund of the hospital would pay the
medical bills, the family only needing to take responsibility for
some other matters: the team would need four pints of blood for
the operation to go ahead and mobilizing this was to be the family's first obligation. Though in development, no reliable machine
was yet ready to take over the work of a person's heart and lungs.
Instead, the family would also need to find an able-bodied adult
with the same blood group who was willing to be a party to the
operation and use his own body to support Mickey's circulation
while the surgeon was operating inside his heart. Problematically,
Mickey's blood group was AB negative – by some margin the
rarest – and neither his parents nor any of his extended family had
the same group.

But Litchfield, Minnesota epitomized 'small town America'
and Litchfield looked after its own. There follows a story of a
human-sized community playing to its strengths. Newsletters and
dinners alerted people to Mickey's situation. The Catholic Church
worked through the Knights of Columbus, the veterans through
the Veterans of Foreign Wars and the district Red Cross organized
blood drives. A local man and father of three got a call out of the
blue. The man's dog-tag data was still on file after his service in the
Second World War and on the telephone was an American Legion
commander. The bizarre proposition was that the man submit to
surgery so that his heart and lungs could support another man's
child while the boy's heart was opened for a life-saving operation.
After meeting Mickey's family and the Minnesota surgeon, and
after the risks and substantial uncertainties had been explained,
Howard Holtz stepped up 'because he hoped someone else would
do the same for his kids if they were sick'. His brother Vernon also
offered. Despite his restrictions, Mickey was a happy-go-lucky kid

who would have learned little of the plans. His mother can only have been grateful; she had enough to do to keep the show on the road at home and organize friends and relatives to look after the other boys. A priest visited.

Underlining the solemnity of the journey, on 24 August 1954 his estranged father turned up to drive Mickey and his mother to the University of Minnesota Heart Hospital in Minneapolis. They would have been an eye-catching group. Mickey, aged eleven and a half but the size of an eight-year-old, wore jeans and check shirt, his parted hair stiff with Butch Wax. Even if trying not to stare, what nobody could quite ignore were his purplish-blue lips and improbably grey complexion, and the way he crouched on a seat with his knees up to his chin.

The hospital had opened only three years previously, long and low with sharp corners, a homage to red brick. Anyone who has themselves paused to take a deep breath on entering a major chil-dren's hospital will recognize the inextricable emotions of hope and fear as you cross the threshold. Upstairs, a forty-bed ward with babies and children, some in for tests, others for surgery, heart problems, leukaemia and infections – a heavy workload with many children likely to die. Down the hall, a ward with thirty patients, some confined to iron lungs; this was the era of the last American polio epidemic. The nurses, who wore white caps on their heads, starched white dresses and thick-soled white shoes, were stern and terribly busy. Visiting hours were strictly enforced: 2–4 p.m. and 6–8 p.m. Toddlers feeling abandoned would be wailing, often tied by their legs to their cribs. Forlorn children would rock themselves to sleep. Offsetting this grim atmosphere was a playroom with a sand-table where children could make mud-pies.

Mickey spent a few days in hospital being checked out. He was weighed, had an electrocardiogram, X-rays, blood and urine tests. Already an object of fascination, many young doctors vis-ited to examine the 'Tet up for surgery'. Before the operation, one of the surgeons – a Dr Lillehei – came to greet him; other patients remember this man as the only doctor who took the trouble to talk to children directly. The AB-negative volunteer blood donors turned up at the hospital the night before the operation to give their pints of fresh blood, and Howard Holtz was admitted and ready.

On the morning of surgery, Mickey was trussed up in a cotton sheet and wheeled down long, bright corridors to a busy operating room. He was helped onto one of the operating tables – still vaguely awake – and a blood pressure cuff wound around his arm. Some local anaesthetic was injected around his inner ankle. A surgeon exposed the big vein that runs there and inserted a chunky metal needle. Because their oxygen levels are so precarious, putting blue children to sleep safely is quite a challenge, and the anaesthetist was loath to do this until a good drip was in place. But when all was set and after a few reassuring words, a mask went over Mickey's face and he drifted off. The anaesthetist prised Mickey's mouth open to insert an instrument to pull his tongue forward and slipped a tube right down his throat, past his vocal cords and down into his windpipe. Mickey breathed on, each breath shifting air through a black rubber bag next to the anaesthetist's hand; now the operation could start.

Observers in the dome above saw Howard being moved onto another operating table and more surgeons arriving and scrubbing up. One team attended to Howard while the other painted Mickey's chest with brown antiseptic and covered him head to toe in green sheets, leaving only a rectangular area framing his chest on which the spotlight was focused. An experienced surgical onlooker would have been struck by the curiosity of having two tables in a single overcrowded operating room and the uncommon spectacle of the two surgeons, Drs Varco and Lillehei, on either side of the main table, working without any sense of rank, each dissecting or stitching what was most readily accessible from his side of the table. One visitor remarked, 'It was impossible to see who was doing what, as there were four hands working in unity. It was extremely interesting to watch.' They proceeded to make the most immense incision – armpit to armpit – aiming between ribs and below the nipples, using a saw across the sternum. Like a needlewoman anticipating seams, one surgeon made little nicks in the skin to guide the matching-up of the edges at the end of the operation. After controlling bleeding vessels, the child's chest was opened up like a clamshell to reveal heart and lungs; huge metal retractors were positioned to keep the field of view clear. With his lungs open to the air, Mickey could no longer breathe for himself and the anaesthetist took over this responsibility by squeezing the black rubber bag.

The heart and the vessels coming in and out of it were exposed, preparing the field for the plumbing that would permit the surgeons to open Mickey's heart without prejudicing the rest of his body. On the adjacent operating table, the other team was preparing the main vein and artery at the top of Howard Holtz's right leg, slipping a plastic tube into each. The tube in the donor's artery was connected to another and fed backwards into Mickey's main artery; it would provide red, oxygenated blood to Mickey's body when his own heart wasn't pumping. Another tube joined Howard's major vein to the main veins returning to Mickey's heart. Before arrangements were quite complete, Mickey's heart suddenly lost power. As if connecting jump-leads to recharge one car battery from another, the team quickly finalized the 'cross-circulation' plumbing so that Howard's heart and lungs could take on the job of supporting Mickey's brain and body. His heartbeat returned, confirming that the situation was no longer precarious. But this circuit only produced between a sixth and a quarter of Mickey's normal heart output, so it could not be relied on to maintain stability for long. The clock started.

Fixing Fallot's tetralogy has two main steps. The surgeons need to open the heart, find and then close the hole between its two pumping chambers; with the hole closed, the blue and red blood can no longer mix through the gap. They then need to relieve the blockage between the heart and the main lung artery.

With Mickey's circulation served by Howard's heart, immediately in front of the surgeons was Mickey's right ventricle, the part of the heart that pumps blood into the lungs. The heart was still beating feebly when they incised it with a scalpel; as expected in Fallot's tetralogy, the muscle was much thicker than normal. Sucking the blood out from the interior of the cavity exposed the anticipated hole between the pumping chambers; so far so good. The nurse at the table handed six curved needles threaded with heavy black silk, one after another, to the surgeons to stitch the hole closed. Before tying down the last stitch and closing off the deeper left ventricle from the outside air, they filled its cavity with salt solution to avoid the possibility of air being pumped around the circulation when the heart began to beat effectively. The team then needed to core out some muscle that was blocking the way through from the interior of the right ventricle to the main lung artery. They kept the bits to photograph for posterity, knowing that this operation was a first of its kind. The right ventricle was then also filled with saline, the initial incision was closed, the heart allowed to fill and accommodate to its new conditions. The heart took over confidently and the cross-circulation circuit connecting Mickey and Howard was closed off.

'How long?' The heart had been open for eleven and a half minutes. Relief was in the air, but there was still a lot to do. After his leg incisions were closed Howard was the first to wake up and he was wheeled back to his ward. Mickey's chest had to be reconstituted, layer by layer, his skin finally stitched using the marking nicks to line things up. Just before the end of the operation the anaesthetic was lightened so that, when the green drapes came off and Mickey was stirring and gasping for breath, the tube was taken out of his throat, and his lungs and his repaired heart were really on their own. Before leaving the spotlight, the surgeons shook hands over the finished job and went off, each to tackle their next case – perhaps the removal of a gall bladder or a hernia repair.

Mickey woke in a weird environment. His bed was inside a clear plastic oxygen tent, its sides tucked under the mattress, its interior cool and damp. The oxygen was piped in from a tall cylinder by the bed and humidified with ice cubes. When the oxygen tent's opening was unzipped, it usually meant an injection (intramuscular penicillin four times a day) or a blood test (needles blunt from use and reuse). His chest, which had been cranked apart, hurt. Moving hurt, breathing hurt, crying hurt, coughing was all but impossible; post-operative pain relief was not an advanced art. Mickey spent two days in a bay on his own with an experienced nurse all to himself; his parents could only peer in through a window. For two days they couldn't get close enough to see how different he looked.

Back on the main ward, he was still in his tent but beginning to eat and drink. This was a lonely, alienated time as bedbound children were pretty much ignored, apart from doctors' rounds or nurses' checklists involving more needles and prodding. Mobile children would literally run away from nurses who pursued them with injections, immune to negotiations involving cookies or juice. Dressings were a misery. The bandages of the day were made of sticky crepe strapping, the stitches underneath snaggy and sore. But Mickey gradually started moving about, first into a wheelchair, then to the playroom; his wounds healed, he could cough (sort of) and when he could raise his arms almost to shoulder level, he was ready to go home. Before the operation, his dad had offered him 50 cents for each detested needle, but the bill got so great that Mickey accepted a new bike instead.

News was leaked to the press when – three weeks after he first

went into hospital – Mickey returned to Litchfield, as pink as his
brothers and ready to join the mainstream of life, a coast-to-coast
celebrity. The achievement of the open-heart repair of a blue
child was a realization of American virtues: the Minneapolis
Heart Hospital itself had been built by the philanthropic efforts
of the Variety Club and in 1952, President Truman had declared
'war against heart disease' and made federal funding available
for heart research. Here was a dividend that would go down in
world history.

But equally 'it takes a village to raise a child' and Litchfield was
chuffed with what it had achieved; their town was in the national
newspapers. Mickey's celebrity was difficult for his brothers – there
had never before been a new bike in the house, let alone a Labrador
puppy 'won' in a rigged prize draw. They were alert to any whiff of
favouritism from their mother. But over the winter, a new family
normality descended. Mickey had missed a lot of school and with
a bright younger brother snapping at his heels in the class below,
he couldn't afford to be put down a year. That was a struggle. But
at twelve years of age, for the first time in his life his legs could
run when he asked them to. After being excused for years, now
he could be required to shovel snow.

The following year he was back in Minneapolis for a check-up.
Contemporary surgeons, who do not expect to be in and out of
the heart of a child with Fallot's tetralogy within an hour, will
not be surprised that tests showed that the hole in Mickey's heart
had not been *quite* closed nor the blockage under the lung artery
quite relieved. But the imperfections balanced out and his progress
testified to the operation's success. His fame lasted for more than
fifteen minutes. His mother mastered her stage-fright and she and
Mickey did several 'benefit gigs' for the hospital. Somewhere in
the family archive is a photograph of Mickey presenting a cheque
for one million dollars; his operation had been a good investment
for the research fund.

As teenage life supervened, Mickey turned into Mike, had a growth spurt, became a dedicated smoker, developed teen-idol looks, joined a band and found rock and roll. As the boys grew taller than her, their mother's influence waned. Mike was up for an occasional fight, usually with a brother. Through high school he took on jobs that middle-sized kids could do – cleaning in the turkey plant, serving in a gas station, selling candy at baseball matches. He was glad to quit high school when he was eighteen. By that time, music was the constant in his life – he played bass guitar in the Nightbeats, the Embers, the Defiants and most successful of all Shaw-Allen-Shaw, the band that thawed the longstanding tension with his no-longer-little brother. They played Minnesota social halls almost every night for seven years and made two records that are still available on eBay. Mike had enough scars to avoid the Vietnam draft but in his fifties he needed coronary surgery. Over the years he never left the music business, working in music stores, as a booking agent or promoter or band manager. You can look him up in the Minnesota Music Hall of Fame. He married happily and his surgeon attended his twenty-fifth wedding anniversary. He had four kids – all musical – and six grandchildren, none of whom would exist but for his operation. His mother believed in miracles and her son was 'the one' who lived at just the right place at just the right time.

Howard Holtz, the modest man who supported Mike's operation is still alive in his eighties. Sixty years after the operation, I could not persuade him to take any credit and had to turn to other local men for a 'testimonial'. It turns out that what Howard Holtz had done for Mickey was completely in character; he had always 'gone the extra mile' for the citizens of his patch of the Forest City township where he maintained the roads and I had not been the only one to find him so self-effacing. Had there been complications, we trust that Litchfield would have looked after his wife and children. Although Dr Lillehei is often portrayed as the star of the cross-circulation operations, for me the outright hero of the first ever Fallot repair was the donor, Howard Holtz.

★   ★   ★

The repair of Mickey's heart was unquestionably a 'first'. But in the hothouse atmosphere of evolving cardiac surgery, 'first' could mean different things: the first floating of an idea, the first experiment, the first (failed) attempt, the first success, the first published record. In the story of the open-heart repair of 'blue' children this was a 'first success', but other children, adults and many, many animals had died on the way to its achievement.

Before Mickey's operation, surgeons in Toronto had tried to repair the hearts of five children with Fallot's tetralogy. While their hearts were open, their bodies were supported by a pump that circulated the patient's blood through the lungs of four recently killed monkeys to oxygenate it. In London there were two rushed attempts without any machine or cross-circulation at all – just cooling the body in the hope of limiting brain damage. All seven children had died. There may well have been other attempts, but failure and shame were close cousins in the surgical community, so we cannot be certain that every death was made public. Using a parent to support their own sick child's circulation, Lillehei had already had a few successes (and failures) in closing straightforward 'holes in the heart'. But the Minneapolis operation using a donor and cross-circulation had provided the 'first success' in repairing the heart of a blue child.

The proposition that a parent uses their own body to maintain their child's life while the child's heart is opened up has an Old Testament feel about it, perhaps fitting for such a God-like endeavour. But striking though it sounds, cross-circulation was not a new idea in medicine. As soon as surgical techniques were up to the job, experimenters were joining together the circulations of two live animals to help answer questions about how blood carries chemical messages; hormones are an example – manufactured in one place, active in another. In a 'proof of principle' exercise, a surgeon at Johns Hopkins Medical School, Baltimore in 1929 established cross-circulation in over forty pairs of dogs by stitching a large artery of each of a pair of dogs to a large vein of the other. After the operations, the pairs of dogs were lashed together with sticky tape and allowed to wake up, move around, feed and sleep. Most died quickly, the suture lines tearing apart or blocking with a clot, or one dog simply bleeding into the other. But two pairs of animals padded around, their circulations joined, for six days. Pedestrians approaching the campus could not avoid knowing about the experiments; there were anti-vivisection posters in a shop window especially rented by the Society for the Prevention of Cruelty to Animals.

By the 1940s, medical experimenters had moved on to trying to use cross-circulation to help human patients. One option was to mingle the circulations of two patients who each had something to gain – patients with the same blood groups but with different illnesses. A woman who had sudden drug-related bone-marrow failure but whose kidneys were working was paired with a younger woman with kidney failure but good bone-marrow function. The blood tests of each improved, but keeping this up day after day was arduous. All parties decided to abandon the trial after two weeks and both women died.*

A second option was to pair patients, one of whom seemed to have something to gain and the other who seemed to have little to lose. In a Californian hospital in 1949 before the advent of chemotherapy, a three-year-old girl was dying of leukaemia; she was moribund, hard to rouse, on the brink. We know her initials

---

* Not before the woman with marrow failure's kidney was transplanted post-mortem into the renal failure patient. The kidney functioned for a while until she too died from an abscess at the suture line.

were 'J. S.' Someone made an incision to find the big vein in her
right groin and stuck in a fat metal cannula attached to a length of
clear rubber tubing. Bumped up close in the adjacent bed was a
thirty-two-year-old man, himself dying of lung cancer. His right
groin was also exposed and cannulated. The tubings were joined
together with a syringe at the junction and blood was manually
sucked from the child and injected into the man, then vice versa,
again and again. After two hours of cross-circulation, two-thirds of
J.S.'s blood volume had been exchange-transfused and both patients
were terribly uncomfortable, needles in their groins, blood seeping
from their wounds. The child became a bit more alert and her
numbers of leukaemia cells circulating had dropped modestly. Next
time, the man in the next bed was a fifty-one-year-old with cancer
ulcerating his lips, tongue and gums. Little J.S. passed away eleven
days after a third exchange and both men died in their own time;
autopsies showed neither had picked up her leukaemia. Each of
the dying volunteers had signed a consent form confirming that
they had understood that their own deaths might be accelerated
or that they could acquire the child's leukaemia. It is not recorded
what form the dying children's parents signed or even whether they
observed her ordeal. Now that we understand more about leukaemia, we know that the child, her parents, the dying volunteers and
the doctors were all embroiled in a hopeless hope.

A last option was to pair a sick person with a fit volunteer,
putting a healthy body at the service of the ill and dying by joining up their circulations – just as the cardiac surgeons were to do
later. Parents, in particular, were willing to take considerable risks
to help their children: in Italy, mothers shared their circulations
with daughters in an effort to relieve the 'persistent vomiting' of
pregnancy. In the USA, an attempt was made to save a son whose
kidneys had stopped working by using his father's kidneys. But
when the father later died as a result of complications arising from
this procedure, this foreshadowed the criticism that the Minneapolis

team later faced when they publicized their open-heart methods; these were interventions that could produce a 200 per cent
mortality.*

Thus already by the early 1950s it had become clear that the
impending death of a child can make people – parents, doctors
and dying patients – take some very extraordinary decisions. Also,
there was a modest practical experience of cross-circulation to
draw from. In therapeutic terms, the interventions had been largely
ineffective but a lot had been learned about how to do it; a 'blood
transfer apparatus' had even been patented. But matters of optimal
blood-flow rates and oxygen transfer had not been addressed and
for this the Minnesota surgeons went back to the animal lab to
refine the cross-circulation technique so that one set of heart and
lungs could serve two bodies.

In the lab, dogs were chosen because they were cheap and
available in a range of sizes. There the Minneapolis surgeons sorted
out the best tubing (clear hose used for siphoning beer), a method
for matching the flows in and out of the two animals (a pump sold
for use in the milking industry) and a regime for preventing clotting
in the plumbing. Then they would stop one of the dog's hearts
so that it depended on the other dog for a short period. When
the assembly was almost perfected, they were impressed that the
dogs would wake up promptly and seem to behave normally. But
they wanted to be as sure as possible that brain damage was not a
side effect of the set-up. A local cardiologist who trained golden

---

* Robert Liston, a surgeon in pre-anaesthesia, pre-surgical-hygiene London was
later described as 'the fastest knife in the West End'; he held the knife between
his teeth to be better able to use a saw. Unfortunately, during one rushed ampu-
tation he accidentally also amputated the fingers of his assistant and slashed the
coat of a spectator. Patient and assistant subsequently died of gangrene and the
spectator, terrified that it was his own blood on the floor, died of a heart attack
on the spot: an operation with a 300 per cent mortality.

retrievers for hunting offered some of his dogs as subjects; after the cross-circulation experiments, they seemed to remember all their commands. The team also realized that any 'donor' would need to be much larger than the 'recipient' if the donor's lungs were to provide enough oxygen for both bodies while the recipient's heart was open and not working. So once again, sick children were to be the subject of the first human experiments.

The first Minneapolis cross-circulation operation took place in February 1954 and the forty-fifth and last in July 1955. After that, acceptable heart-lung machines had been developed. Forty-three of the operations involved a parent as the blood-group-matched donor. Apart from Mickey Shaw and Howard Holtz, the only other exception was the pairing of a three-year-old boy with a woman prisoner from a local penitentiary.*

Sixteen of the forty-five children died in hospital. One operation, in which a mother was sharing her circulation with her daughter, was halted when horrified spectators in the dome above the operating table saw what nobody on the operating-room floor below had noticed – a column of air being pumped into the mother's circulation through the clear tubing. There was no audio connection between upstairs and downstairs. The mother's heart stopped as the air was pumped through her circulation and the operating room descended into commotion; though she survived, the bubbles that had blocked vessels in her brain left her more childlike than her children.

The audacity and technical achievement of operating inside a child's heart was a godsend to the world of photo-journalism. Sandwiched between an advertisement for cake-mix and another for Fitch's Hair Tonic, *Life* magazine of November 1954 has a

---

* In that era 40 per cent of blood donations in America came from people in correctional facilities: the Minnesota men's prison had a club called the 'Leaky Arm' club.

photo-montage of the whole glorious story: a sick baby, a 'living heart cut open', a husband bending over his wife after her return from the surgery and a final photo of the mother's reward as she cradles her post-operative infant.

When we learn that the daughter of that brain-damaged mother survived to be operated on using a heart-lung machine six years later, we have to wonder if some of the other patients who had died post-operatively might not have been better advised to wait. In principle, there had even been another option for Mickey Shaw. A Blalock shunt operation would at least have made him pinker and given him more energy; such surgery had already been available for almost ten years. This 'shunt' option had been mentioned, but in terms of the research fund financing Mickey's surgery, it was the open heart offer or nothing. For Mickey's parents, their lack of money meant lack of choice.

3
When nothing is done

efore the 1940s, there was no treatment for children born with heart defects and, because their private lives were undocumented, it is difficult to illustrate their destinies. Yet in the first half of the last century there are two people born with heart conditions whose life-stories help us to understand how heart disease curtails the existence of people left unoperated. The only reason we know about them at all is through their biographers – because they became famous before they died. One of these was Dick Ket, later a celebrated artist, born in 1902 with what was almost certainly tetralogy of Fallot, though this was not diagnosed in his lifetime.

Ket was born in Den Helder, a Dutch coastal town that had been going downhill since the eighteenth century. The family later moved to The Hague with his father's job as an army pharmacy assistant. Ket was an only child with a protective mother. He was bullied at school. Delivering medicines around town to help his father, he was slow, puffing and stooping as shoppers overtook him.

He went to art school in Arnhem at the age of twenty and there met teachers who introduced him to the worlds of theosophy and mysticism. These ideas became important to him: perhaps he sensed that his life would be short and could end at any moment. There are many competent sketches of landscapes and townscapes in Dutch collections from his art-school era, along with the first of his self-portraits: one showing a larky young man dressed in a spivvy suit and another, from 1927, in which he is a little more dishevelled but still very much the student.

By the time he was twenty-six, his disability was becoming very limiting; the family had moved and the commute to Arnhem had become intolerable for him. A house was built to his specifications with a ground-floor bedroom and studio, and after 1930 he rarely left home. Largely isolated from the art world, his artistic style matured. In 1932 he painted his girlfriend, Nel Schilt, and they were briefly engaged; although she married someone else a couple of years later, they kept in touch by letter to the end of his life.* He had a one-man exhibition in 1933, which he did not have the strength to attend, and in 1935 won the Queen's gold medal for a self-portrait. But within a year he was struggling even to finish his canvases. He was sometimes in bed for weeks.

Tetralogy is a common diagnosis that sometimes allows blue babies to survive through childhood; it is the condition shared by Mickey Shaw and many of Blalock's patients. Every cell of our bodies needs oxygen, and these patients' cells don't get enough. The less oxygen that is carried in the blood, the bluer, more limited and fatigued the patient will be. Severe lack of oxygen will gradually ruin every organ and tissue: brain, muscle, heart, skin.

As Ket's horizons narrowed, he started to paint the self-portraits for which he became best known. These serve as his completely unsentimental, almost forensic record of how his heart disease was wrecking his body. In his studio with its gloomy, prison-like background – no window, no cosiness – he documented his blue-grey

* Some 450 letters are kept in Royal Library, The Hague.

complexion, his suffused eyes and his rotten gums in meticulous detail. It is as if in his studio mirror we can see his inner state, a sort of anti-hero wedged inside his crumbling physique. He died at home in 1940 at the age of thirty-six – four years before Blalock performed the first shunt operation in North America.

Exhibitions in prestigious museums have been mounted since Ket's death. Most catalogues claim that he would not venture out in his final years because of agoraphobia and paranoia about visitors, but it is at least as plausible that, for the last years of his life, he simply could neither walk beyond his garden gate nor bear to be viewed by sightseers from the land of the well.

★   ★   ★

Before the 1940s the brief lives and inevitable deaths of children were isolated, family affairs. Yet if we want to convey in cold numbers – rather than in stories – what happens to people born with congenital heart disease when nothing is done, we need to look at what happened in a society that kept a careful count of all of its citizens; a society that was stable over many years with little immigration or emigration; a society in which every child's death was fully documented by doctors competent to discriminate the many forms of congenital heart disease – yet one in which no surgery was available that might alter the 'natural history' of the disease.

Such a society existed in Central Bohemia when Czechoslovakia was part of the Eastern Bloc (this area is now in the Czech Republic and is very well served for the treatment of congenital heart disease). In the years from 1952 to 1979, 468,733 babies were born in Central Bohemia. A full autopsy, supervised by a pathologist who specialized in heart malformations, was performed on every child who died before the age of fifteen. This provided 946 well-documented reports, including a reliable diagnosis and the age at which the child died. From this data it is possible to see the typical age at which a person born with each of the common congenital heart diseases would die. It is hard to see how such a study could ever be repeated.

In the Bohemian study, children with heart problems were at the greatest risk of dying soon after birth: 10 per cent of all deaths in childhood from heart disease happened in the very first week of life. After one month, 30 per cent of babies with Transposition of the Great Arteries had died, along with 80 per cent of those with Hypoplastic Left Heart Syndrome, 50 per cent of those with Total Anomalous Pulmonary Venous Drainage and 40 per cent of babies with pulmonary atresia. (Sorry for the jargon here, but we will meet and understand more about the particular problems later; they represent varieties of 'critical' congenital heart disease.) All these diagnoses involve some abnormality that makes the transition at birth to lung-breathing life very problematic. No baby in any of these groups survived to the age of two.

In the report, 60 per cent of babies born with Fallot's tetralogy – Dick Ket's disease – lived to their first birthday, 23 per cent to their tenth and only 4 per cent to their fifteenth; he was a rare survivor into adulthood.

The commonest of all anomalies among the Bohemian babies was a hole between the pumping chambers of the heart – Ventricular Septal Defect (VSD). One in five babies with a significant VSD died in the first year of life, but the others survived childhood. Unfortunately this did not necessarily mean that they survived unscathed. As we've seen, Ket's health inexorably deteriorated throughout his life. Children with a VSD take a different course; if they survive babyhood, some will be tolerably well for many years but may yet run into trouble.

To illustrate, we know of another famous but fated victim of untreated congenital heart disease: the legendary Indian film actress Madhubala. She is to Bollywood what Marilyn Monroe is to Hollywood, an icon who died young. In her time, even an American film magazine called her 'the biggest star in the world'.*

Born in 1933, as a child Madhubala† was a cute singer and dancer, and her family gravitated towards Bombay, famous for its film industry. When she was only nine years old, her pushy father landed her a small part in a Bombay 'talkies' movie. From that debut to her death, she brought in most of the family's income. Her first big break came in *Neel Kamal* when the director's wife, who was scheduled to play the lead role, died after filming had started. Madhubala knew the dialogue and stepped into the part, becoming a Bollywood heroine at the age of thirteen. At sixteen she was dominating the film posters for a reincarnation thriller, *Mahal*, which was a huge box-office hit that made her a superstar. She was bright and bubbly, and if she knew she was ill she was telling nobody.

During a shoot in 1954, when she was twenty, she coughed up some blood; she went straight back to filming. In 1957, she fainted on set. Nobody had previously recognized that she had a VSD. Her heart and lungs had accommodated the situation for twenty-four years, but a tipping point had been reached. By now she was going visibly blue, at first intermittently, later constantly. For the first time, a doctor diagnosed her underlying problem and knew that things were about to go downhill badly. He could suggest no treatment other than bed rest, but Madhubala was not ready to believe that she was sick and again resumed work. The movies had gone into colour, but lipstick and nail varnish were sufficient disguise.

Her fans were unaware of her medical problems, privacy being

---

* 'The biggest star in the world – and she is not even in Beverly Hills', said in the American magazine *Theatre Arts* in 1952. The black-and-white pictures in *Life* magazine are especially wonderful. Madhubala's father vetoed the subsequent approaches from Hollywood.
† Actually she was born Mumtaz Begum. Madhubala (literally 'Honey Belle') was her screen name.

very much part of her mystique; when she occasionally went out to
the cinema with her sisters, she wore a burqa. These were the days
when Indian censors banned the on-screen kiss, so impropriety
was never on the surface. This allowed her fans to speculate about
her love life, as her suitors were many and not so reticent. After
breaking up with Dilip Kumar, her leading man in several films, on
the rebound Madhubala married another big star, Kishore Kumar.
This was in 1960, Madhubala was twenty-seven and news about
the early open-heart operations in the USA was out. Though it
is never mentioned in her biopics, the Indian doctors must have
briefed her against pregnancy. Madhubala and her new husband
travelled to London, perhaps for a second opinion, perhaps to find
out if money could buy surgery. Instead, the English doctor told
her that she did not have long to live and almost certainly strongly
vetoed a pregnancy, which would typically be lethal for a mother
with an untreated large VSD.

Madhubala was now 'damaged goods'. On their return to India,
Kishore dumped her in a house with a maid and a driver and rarely
visited or even took her calls. No longer cinematic hot property, with
no reason to dress up and detached even from her family, Madhubala
became depressed, spending her days watching her own films from
her sickbed. A sister recorded that, towards the end, 'every four to five
hours she had to be given oxygen or else would get breathless'. She
died in 1969 at the age of thirty-six. On her father's insistence, her
personal diaries were buried with her. Her marble tomb in Mumbai
was demolished in 2010 on the orders of the Wahhabi sect administering the cemetery, but her fans still maintain a Facebook page.

★　★　★

Why did a hole in Madhubala's heart cause so much trouble for
her – and so late in life? To understand, we'll need an account of
the 'circulation' – the plumbing of the heart and the way the blood
circulates through it. If this is something you already understand,

this is a good time to skip ahead – especially if you are squeamish about mixed metaphors.

A baby's heart is about the size of a baby's fist; your heart about the size of your fist. The heart muscle squeezes, much like a fist would, and squirts blood out through pipes with each beat. After each squeeze it relaxes and re-fills with more blood. You cannot tell much about its internal architecture from looking at the outside of the heart, though you can see two pipes coming out of the top – one goes to the lungs (the pulmonary artery: 'pulmonary' meaning 'pertaining to the lungs' and 'artery' meaning 'vessel carrying blood away from the heart') and the other to the body (the aorta). If you look carefully, you may notice that the upper and lower portions of the heart are beating at the same rate but at slightly different times and that the lower portion of the heart seems to be doing most of the work. (Medical students remember the cadence of these coordinated beats as 'lub-dub'.) As you look at the heart in situ, you cannot actually see the pipes (veins) that are arriving into the back of the heart receiving blood from the lungs and body.

A diagram shows the internal structure of the heart better (there are several diagrams in the Appendix, on page 293). It consists of four chambers; the two upper (atria) are floppy and accommodate the blood that arrives continuously and the two lower chambers (ventricles) are muscular and pump it out again intermittently. We call the collecting and pumping chambers serving the lungs the right atrium and right ventricle; those serving the body are the left atrium and left ventricle. (Though we label the chambers 'right' and 'left', in reality the heart is a 3-dimensional structure and usually the right ventricle is also in 'front' of the left ventricle.)* There is

---

* Exasperatingly, in complex congenital heart disease, the right atrium may well be on the left or there might even be two left atria and no right atrium. Learning the language that permits us to specify heart structures unambiguously is a tough part of a specialist's training – like learning a dialect that few understand.

a wall (septum) between the right and left atria (atrial septum) and another between the right and left ventricles (ventricular septum); in a normal heart, there are no holes in these walls. In the floor of each atrium is a trapdoor (valve) through which the waiting blood can fall as soon as the ventricle below has relaxed and allowed the trapdoor to open. These valves – along with the pulmonary valve at the junction of the right ventricle and pulmonary artery and the aortic valve at the junction of left ventricle and aorta – help to maintain the one-way flow of blood around the circulation.

When we talk of 'the circulation', we are describing how the blood goes endlessly around in two loops – a schematic would look much like a child's racing-car track that is configured as a figure-of-eight. The two parts of the circuit serve the lungs and the body. In the standard-issue heart, the lung and body circuits are joined in a simple sequence, but we will see that the plumbing of congenital heart disease can be complicated by all sorts of possible short-cuts, unconventional connections, blockages and leaks inside and outside the heart. But with or without congenital heart disease, if the movement of blood through the body circuit falls below a certain threshold, or if the blood in that circuit contains insufficient oxygen, you die.

Blood has many jobs, but its most pressing task is to transport the oxygen that it picks up as it passes through the lungs and deliver it to every cell of your body. It changes colour at different points on its journey. As it leaves the lungs, blood is bright red because haemoglobin, the amazing molecule packed inside the blood cells of animals, changes colour depending on how much oxygen it is carrying. Normally, this red blood is then pumped around the body, where working cells unload the oxygen and use it to generate energy. Depleted of oxygen, the blood returns to the heart looking dark, more purplish – the colour of blood in a blood transfusion bag. If a child looks blue, it is because the blood running around their body doesn't contain enough oxygen; their energy levels will be correspondingly poor. A child might be blue because insufficient blood is reaching their lungs, or because the blue and red blood are mixing up somewhere (probably inside an unusual heart) or because an abnormal connection means that blue and red blood are streaming unfavourably – at worst, the blue blood might be piped towards the body and red blood to the lungs.

The heart is at the hub of the body and lung circuits; it accelerates the blood as it passes through, giving it enough shove to get it around the next part of its journey. If we think of the circulation in terms of traffic-flow around the child's racing track, the track runs from the heart around the lungs and back to the heart, then out around the body and back to the heart and so on continuously – heart-lung-heart-body-heart-lung . . . Squeezing simultaneously, the right ventricle pushes it through the lungs, the left pushes it around the body.

If there are no short-cuts in the circuit, the total amount of blood flowing through the lungs must necessarily match that flowing through the body. In the lung circuit, blood is normally very free-flowing because its roads (blood vessels) are numerous and broad. This means that the right ventricle does not need to generate much force to drive blood through the lungs. The bulk of the heart's muscle is in the wall of the left ventricle, because pushing blood through the body involves much more work – the road network is more extensive and in many regions the minor roads are very narrow. In the normal heart, beat for beat, the left ventricle works about thirty times harder than the right ventricle. We usually measure your 'body' blood pressure with a cuff around your arm; if the reading is, say, 120/80 mmHg* in your arm, it is probably about 20/10 in your lung artery.

* 120 is the highest pressure recorded in the cycle, 80 the lowest. mmHg are the units the pressure is measured in (the height of a column of mercury in millimetres).

Blockages can occur in the system and, as we know, traffic backs up behind a hold-up. The obstruction might be a motorway accident where four lanes are reduced to one – a 'local blockage' – perhaps the pulmonary valve might not open easily, forcing the right ventricle to generate a higher pressure to get blood past the stiff valve. Alternatively, a busy road might taper down into little lanes with a smaller capacity – a 'diffuse blockage'; the disease of 'high blood pressure' or 'hypertension' is like this. The small and medium-sized vessels in the body become narrower, which means that the left ventricle needs to work harder, and generate a higher pressure (perhaps 200/100 mmHg) to push the blood around the body. We will see that high blood pressure can happen in the lung circuit too (this is called pulmonary hypertension). As we move on to the more exotic circuits of congenital heart disease, it is worth remembering that if there is a diversion available, many cars grid-locked in traffic will use it to avoid a bottleneck. In the same way, flowing blood will tend to take the path of least resistance.

Now we have enough background to understand Madhubala's life story. She was born with a big hole in the wall between her ventricles – a VSD. The presence of the hole gave the blood in both ventricles a free choice of routes out of the heart. Each blood cell (each car) could either leave through the aorta, and go to the body, or it could leave through the pulmonary artery and go to the lungs. In early childhood, with each squeeze, most of the blood favoured the 'path of least resistance' and flooded out to the lungs – as though traffic had found it much easier to drive through the lungs than having to drive all around the body. Technically, we call this choice of direction of blood flow a 'left to right shunt'. As a young child, it is likely that there was three or four times more blood going through Madhubala's lungs than through the whole of her body. The pressure in the lung circuit would have been very high – with a hole of this size, the pressures in the two ventricles must have equalized. If her body blood pressure was 100/70, the pressure in her lung artery was probably about 100/20 – far higher than normal. As a young child Madhubala probably had a loud murmur, a noise that could be heard if you'd pressed a stethoscope to her heart, caused by the huge volume of blood rushing across the hole and out to the lungs. Many babies falter in this phase; all the extra blood makes their lungs stiff and the lungs' sogginess makes the child prone to chest infections. Breathing is hard work, and sucking and breathing at the same time is a struggle, so these babies often feed poorly. In the Central Bohemia study, 20 per cent of babies born with large VSDs died before their first birthday. We do not know if Madhubala was a worry to her family as a baby.

Then, during the first years of Madhubala's life, the excessive pressure gradually started to ruin her lungs. In the same way that pressure of traffic ravages tarmac, the too-fast, high-pressure flow stripped away fragments of the delicate lining of the lung's blood vessels and a cycle of repetitive damage and healing started. The structure of lung arteries has not evolved to withstand high pressures, and sections of the walls of small arteries started to bulge and blow out, giving way like old bicycle tyres. Little bursts and small bleeds distorted and blocked nearby vessels. As damaged vessels in the lung bed become clogged up, it becomes more difficult for the blood to flow through them. In the short term, this can seem to help. As the lung circuit becomes more damaged, less blood takes this 'path of least resistance' and the 'left to right shunt' decreases. The child has 'pulmonary vascular disease'. It is perhaps counter-intuitive, but children at this stage often have no symptoms and hardly any murmur; this has usually happened by the time they are about five years old. Enough blood is getting through their lungs to keep them pink, their hearts are adapted to the situation and typically their activity levels are similar to their classmates'. For them, childhood is often a sort of 'honeymoon period'.

Unfortunately, the lung vessel destruction continues invidiously. If the little blow-outs in vessel walls spill into the nearby

small airways, the patient may cough up the blood. As the damage gets even worse, a 'tipping point' occurs: the lungs are so
blocked that the 'path of least resistance' for blood in both ventricles is to go around the body. Now, the blue blood that should
be going through the lungs to pick up oxygen reaches the body
instead, and the person becomes visibly blue. We say that the 'shunt
has reversed' – now it operates 'right to left'. The name for this
state is 'Eisenmenger's syndrome'.* When this first happened to
Madhubala, she was fainting with little effort.

Madhubala's health problems began in late teenage life and
she died at the age of thirty-six. This is typical of what happens
to children born with a big hole who do not have surgery, but
who manage to survive the soggy-lung phase often seen in early
childhood. In Madhubala's day, bed-rest and oxygen were the only
treatments available. By the time a child has pulmonary vascular
disease, her lung-blood vessels are irreparably damaged and it is too
late to close the hole in the heart; she would die at surgery. We
have to operate when the child is much younger.

In the year 2012–2013, 330 simple VSDs were closed in
young children in the UK, and, although two children died
post-operatively, many of the other 328 have probably been saved
from Madhubala's fate. But before we think that closing all these
VSDs in babyhood means that Eisenmenger's syndrome is con-
signed to history, let me introduce you to Sophie.

Sophie and I made a date to meet, gossiping in a classy café
like any two women. She is tall with glossy, dark hair and pale
skin, beautifully dressed. You might call her elegant but there is
something a little edgy, a bit 'goth' about her. She takes the comment 'Like your lipstick' as a compliment though she doesn't wear
any. Likewise, 'Why does someone like you only work part time?'

---

* The phenomenon of blood flow flipping direction in the face of increasing
resistance in the lungs can happen in anomalies other than VSD.

calls up a flicker of pride because she loves to pass as normal. But being twenty-something and not able to remember staying out after 10 p.m., to be watching your friends have babies, to live determinedly for today while slapping down daydreams about the future is a very tough script. Sophie is a contemporary young woman with Eisenmenger's syndrome.

Sophie had a murmur and was seen by cardiac specialists when she was six months old; they diagnosed a VSD. As a young child, she was never dreadfully ill, but somehow the operation that she needed as an investment for her future was never offered, and by the time she was five years old investigations showed it was too late.

She sailed through primary school and went on to be a level-headed grammar-school girl. Sophie took herself out of sport when she was fourteen because she was slower than the others, and hated it anyway. She got good grades and at seventeen was in her final year of school, heading for university. Then, out of the blue, while sitting on the sofa she got a terrible thudding in her chest and nearly blacked out. An ambulance was called, but the hospital quickly diagnosed a 'panic attack' and sent her home. These 'swimmy feelings' began to come frequently, so she did not dare leave the house. Her doctors and school were content with the label of 'stress' in a middle-class, high-achieving girl facing exams; they even briefly persuaded her family of the diagnosis. But Sophie knew there was something really wrong and not being taken seriously was doing her head in. She drank, she got weepy and was excluded from school for non-attendance. Her university applications were never completed. A psychiatrist put her on anti-psychotic medication.

After six months she had a 'mind over matter' turnaround. Over the telephone, a specialist nurse told her she had Eisenmenger's syndrome, a diagnosis nobody had ever mentioned to her before. 'Whatever,' she said, and went out with her mates. (She later Googled 'Eisenmenger's' but what she saw made her panicky and she stopped.) Her friends went off to university and she found a desk job. At work, when she was twenty-one, she coughed up some blood. It took some time for the receiving hospital to understand why a 'fit' young woman would do this, but she eventually reached a specialist hospital where they recognized the problem. She has subsequently had a mini-stroke, weakness starting in her hand, her leg crumpling; in hospital a brain scan showed that a clot that almost certainly started in a vein had shot across the hole into her brain. She recovered well but has been on anti-clotting medicines ever since. While many of her friends are having babies, at every clinic visit she is reminded to use two forms of contraception rather than risk pregnancy. Pregnancy is very risky for women with Eisenmenger's syndrome as placentas make huge demands for blood to nourish the fetus. As more blood is diverted to the placenta, less blood goes through the lungs, so the mother can become dangerously blue. Some friends have offered to be surrogate mothers for Sophie – but she knows she has not got the energy for a baby.

In her twenties, Sophie works part-time, arriving home exhausted. She is good at online computer games, sees friends a couple of times per week and on a bad day can't manage a flight of stairs. Her outlook is not as bad as Madhubala's; there are now some drugs that can help people with pulmonary hypertension, and heart and lung transplantation is a theoretical possibility. But Sophie's trust in doctors is at rock-bottom.

We might now call Sophie's situation tragic, not because we necessarily expect all babies born with congenital heart disease to survive, but because we expect them all at least to be offered treatment if they need it. But heart surgery for children is an expensive enterprise and worldwide not all can afford it. Estimates suggest that 655,000 children are born globally every year with problems that would qualify for an operation if they were born in contemporary Europe, the USA or Australia. In practice, only a quarter of children worldwide actually receive surgery. The lifespan of the other 490,000 will be consistent with their diagnosis. Collectively the burden of congenital heart disease around the world remains enormous. In Africa, for example, there is only one cardiac surgeon for every 38 million people, compared to one for every 3.5 million in North America and Europe and one for every 25 million in Asia. This means that there must be many Madhubalas and Dick Kets and Sophies living in Africa – adults who are not wage earners, unable to contribute to their families.

Can anything be done? Until basic-level health services improve considerably, it is hard to see how most babies born with the anomalies that kill soon after birth can be saved; their chance of surviving even to diagnosis is very low. But the Central Bohemia study suggests that 80 per cent of babies with a VSD and half of those with tetralogy will reach their second birthday and, in principle they could benefit from an operation. The treatment of congenital heart disease will always be expensive and arguably not a priority in resource-poor countries. However, the cost of lifetime treatment of an African baby with HIV infection would be a comparable amount to closing a VSD – and although closure of a VSD is effectively curative, it is universal HIV treatment that is the priority healthcare goal for many countries.

International charities have brought third-world children to first-world hospitals for surgery. In England in 1996, the 'Chain of Hope' brought seven-year-old Arnaud Wambo from Cameroon for an operation. To help publicize the charity, Princess Diana watched the surgery and the media watched her.* These days, 'medical missions' sponsored by individuals and companies and staffed by volunteer surgeons, cardiologists, technicians and nurses go out for a couple of weeks at a time to perform operations in the larger

---

* This was at the time of her divorce from Prince Charles and the press's fault-finding was at its height – they famously carped at the mascara she was wearing.

cities of the children's own countries. If you want to transform the future of a poor child in the developing world, you need only raise the cost of a modest second-hand car,* and a travelling team will perform the operation on your behalf.

* The Chain of Hope 'Sponsor a Child' arrangement suggests that £5,000, $7,500 or €6,400 will cover the costs of a child's heart operation.

4
Birth was almost the death of him

To be a much-wanted first child should be a great start in life, and initially this is how it seemed when Adam was born. Some delivery-room photos were taken, he was discharged quickly from hospital and it was not long before his extended family was demanding baby-viewings. Although his parents, Majda and Nadir, were not quite comfortable with Adam's colour, it is easy to reassure first-time parents – the visiting midwife said it was just the winter light and 'new mummy anxiety'.

Adam was eight days old on New Year's Eve. His parents had intended to stay with relatives overnight to celebrate, but the baby was not feeding well so they took their worries home. Adam showed no interest in sucking and was making little grunting noises as he breathed. As anxiety mounted, Nadir cradled the tense little bundle while Majda rooted out the midwife's phone number. As Nadir looked down at his new son, the baby's urgent gasping stopped, and his father had to lurch forward to scoop him up as he collapsed like a noodle. Adam was not breathing. Call for an ambulance.

Bubbling up from a long-ago scuba-training class came some instructions: breathe gently into the mouth. The emergency services call-taker stayed on the line: 'Is the chest going up and down?', 'Can you feel a heartbeat?', 'Keep going; help is on its way.' And it was. In less than five minutes, a man wearing a motorbike helmet was sprinting up the stairs. As they worked together on the baby, they heard the ambulance's siren overshooting the driveway and Majda had to struggle out into the snowy countryside to flag it down.

The arriving crew had a pretty comprehensive skillset; a tube was put down Adam's throat, into his windpipe and attached to a squeeze-bag so his lungs could be breathed with oxygen. Compressing his chest had restored some sort of heartbeat and the casualty department of the nearest hospital was only ten min-utes away.

Adam was still precarious as he was handed over to the wait-ing team. Resuscitation drugs are generally given through plastic cannulas that someone, somehow, has poked into a vein. Even in the best circumstances this can be tricky, but this was a small baby whose little body was being rocked by the breathing-bag and occasional chest compressions so the drugs were injected straight into Adam's bone marrow through a fat needle puncturing his shin-bone.

Some sort of stability was achieved. It was clear that Adam was blue and that his lungs were very stiff. In a baby born at term, this pointed to a heart problem that would need urgent surgical atten-tion, so the next step was to find a specialist unit with an available bed on New Year's Eve – and another team to transport him there with all the technology to which he was now attached: monitors, drips, a ventilator.

Blue lights, snow and traffic. The ambulance had to stop on the threshold of the receiving hospital; the incubator was opened and more chest compressions delivered. By the time Adam's parents tumbled out of the ambulance and into the arms of the intensive care staff, they were prostrate with stress and fatigue. A cardiac diagnosis was quickly confirmed. A surgeon had been re-routed from his party plans. He explained the nature of the problem to Adam's parents; the veins returning blood from the lungs to the heart were wrongly connected and obstructed. The solution was simple but not easy. Adam was heading into the operation already very ill and, in such a situation, the surgeon would expect three out of ten babies to die post-operatively. But Adam's parents had no difficulty believing that without surgery there was no chance at all; their baby was operated on that night.

Adam was a 'blue baby' but the cause of his blueness was different from that of Mickey Shaw or indeed any of Blalock's patients. His heart was built nearly perfectly, with two collecting, two pumping chambers, and two main arteries, but there was one problem: the veins carrying the blood back to the heart from his lungs had joined up wrongly. All the red blood returning from his lungs arrived in the right (wrong) atrium, where it met all the blue blood from his body.* This meant that the right side of the heart and the lungs quickly swelled up with all the extra blood. Fortunately a newborn's circulation takes a few days to adapt after birth from its in-the-womb arrangements, otherwise Adam's circuit would have been rapidly fatal as the right heart became overloaded and the left heart and body emptied of blood.

In the womb, by three weeks after conception (baby the size of a sesame seed), beating heart cells are discernible. By six weeks after conception (baby the size of a broad bean), the heart and main blood vessels are basically built and providing all the circulation to the growing fetus. Thus by six weeks after conception, if arteries are joined up incorrectly, if a valve has not formed, if veins are connected to the wrong chambers, there is no going back.

---

* This is called Total Anomalous Pulmonary Venous Drainage/Connection or TAPVD/C.

A fetus's nourishment and oxygen come exclusively from the placenta. With no air to breathe, unborn lungs are useless; their blood vessels are squashed, restricting the free-flow of blood through them. Thus a fetus's circulation needs to operate differently from an air-breathing newborn's. The blood can – indeed must – bypass the lungs and deliver much of the heart's output to the vessels in the baby's umbilical cord and placenta. Fetal blood takes advantage of one shortcut inside (a hole between the collecting chambers) and another outside the heart (a vessel called the ductus which joins the lung artery directly to the body artery as it heads down towards the placenta). Like traffic faced with a choice of alternative routes, blood leaving the right heart tends to take the path of least resistance and rushes down to the free-flowing placenta rather than losing speed through the gridlocked lungs.

It is the presence of these 'short-cuts' in an unborn baby's heart that permits them to thrive in the womb even if there are heart malformations that will later prove devastating. Taking advantage of the hole between the atria and/or the duct joining the lung and body arteries, a heart that is abnormally built can continue to deliver enough blood to the placenta despite blockages, missing components or oddly connected arteries or veins. Babies with even serious congenital heart disease are typically born near term with a respectable birth-weight. But these communications are programmed to close once a baby is born, even when this is the last thing a baby with an abnormal heart needs.

After birth, new constraints kick in quickly. Adam made a first cry, the midwife clamped and cut his umbilical cord and he was irrevocably committed to breathing on his own. As his lungs expanded, their vessels began to accommodate more flow from the heart and the blood picked up the oxygen successfully, but the blood then arrived back in the right (wrong) atrium and was destined to be pumped back to the lungs again; so Adam had an immediate problem. Fortunately, the hole between the collecting chambers persists for a while, so when blood started backing up in the overloaded lung circuit, some could pour through the hole to be pumped around the body. This means that the body of a baby with Adam's condition receives a mixture of blue and red blood; we have to wonder why Adam was not more ill before his discharge, and indeed why nobody spotted that he was more blue than he should have been.

In practice, newborns are quite comfortable with oxygen levels that would terrify a doctor looking after an adult – babies have spent the past nine months well adapted to low amounts of circulating oxygen. Even the blueness in newborn 'blue babies' is rarely very noticeable; it's more of a 'not-quite-pink' quality. This goes some way to explaining why more than one in four blue babies leaves hospital after birth having been 'passed as normal' by three separate screening tests: first, an ultrasound scan of the heart before the baby is born, then the quick assessment in the delivery room, and finally the postnatal 'check-up', usually carried out before a baby leaves hospital. The key aim of screening tests it to recognize problems before symptoms cause real trouble, averting the sort of dramatic deterioration that seriously threatened Adam's life.

In the UK, almost all mothers are offered a scan at about twenty weeks of pregnancy and most take up the offer, if only to get a glimpse of their baby. These scans are carried out in the maternity hospital to check the growth of the baby and the position of the placenta, and to inspect limbs, face, spine, brain, kidneys and heart for abnormalities. Getting a complete set of pictures of a baby lying in an awkward position is really tricky, though the sonographer will usually manage to see the heart. Her task is to notice anything unusual, perhaps an asymmetry or a strikingly bright area that might be a clue to an abnormality. If there is any concern, the pregnant woman will then need to travel to a clinic where a specialist can make a fuller diagnosis and answer the torrent of questions that follow any bad news. Currently in the UK, about

45 per cent of babies needing surgery for congenital heart disease in the first year of life have the diagnosis made before they are born; in the USA, it is closer to 15 per cent.

For those that remain undiagnosed, the next opportunity to notice a problem is in the delivery room. At one minute and again at five minutes after birth, every baby is given an APGAR score in case they need urgent medical attention. Virginia Apgar was an anaesthetist, but many hospital staff remember: Appearance, Pulse, Grimace, Activity, Respiration. Staff check whether the child is breathing, moving, crying, has a reasonable heart rate or looks pale or blue. A score of 0–2 on each element when added up gives a score from 0–10; a score below 3 has staff calling for urgent help. Delivery is stressful for babies and it is actually unusual for a baby to have an APGAR score of 10 out of 10; even at five minutes it is common for babies not to be definitely pink. The APGAR score is not a good screen for heart disease.

There is generally a slightly more leisurely check before the baby goes home. Parents will themselves have noticed any obvious abnormalities – a cleft lip, extra fingers or toes, wonky ears or some genital anomalies. Using a checklist, staff examine the baby from head to toe looking for more subtle oddities, including murmurs or weak pulses or a problematic colour, and get help if anything is worrying. Nevertheless, about 40 per cent of babies with very serious congenital heart disease still leave hospital with their problems unrecognized, having been passed as normal in all these tests. Their disease will go on to declare itself through symptoms which can evolve rapidly – as happened to Adam. Undoubtedly some suspicious signs are missed, perhaps through staff inexperience or pressure of time, but mothers with well-looking babies are often discharged within hours of birth when the diagnostic clues may not have even emerged.

Measuring every baby's oxygen saturation with a machine before they go home does pick up some blue babies that would be missed even by a competent clinical eye. But for every baby whose heart problem is correctly diagnosed in this way, about sixteen other babies' oximeter readings will produce 'false alarms'; these babies are not perfectly pink at the time of the test, though their hearts are normal and they will pink-up later when their lungs dry out. An early diagnosis can avoid catastrophic deterioration for an affected baby; but these results can also cause unnecessary alarm and extra testing for sixteen times more families whose baby's oximeter readings are only temporarily low.

Despite the screening failures and his shocking collapse at home, Adam came through. Of course, he remembers nothing, but his parents recall the ordeal in excruciating detail. I last saw him when he was five years old, showing his little brother how to hang upside down from a trapeze in the family's garden.

★ ★ ★

Another couple, another first pregnancy. Rajni and Ian were looking forward to getting a view of their baby when they took time off work to attend the ultrasound scan at twenty weeks. Chatting to the sonographer, they were delighted to hear that the baby was a boy. The final views were taking a long time and the sonographer sent them off to walk about and perhaps have some chocolate to stimulate the baby, in the hope that he might move around to an easier scanning position. Returning, she was still not happy and neither was her supervisor. Ominously, Rajni and Ian were sent upstairs to the Fetal Medicine Unit and a specialist who scanned the baby was still doubtful. They were told to come back for another scan after the weekend.

Rajni and Ian went home and hung around each other with a sense of doom and foreboding. On the Monday, the same doctor repeated the scan and was sure of the problem. Like Adam's, this baby's heart was built perfectly but for the fact that the arteries leaving the heart were the wrong way round, each coming off the wrong pumping chamber.* While this wouldn't matter much in the womb where the placenta was providing the oxygen, after birth things would go wrong quite quickly. With this unpromising arrangement, all the red blood coming back from the lungs would be pumped out to the lungs again and all the blue blood returning from the body would be pumped back out to the body. After birth, the baby would not be able to leave hospital without a major operation to reconnect the arteries correctly. And he might not survive that operation. At the end of the conversation, the specialist suggested that they consider whether they wanted to carry on with the pregnancy, assuring them that they would have help whatever they decided.

They thought about an abortion, but not for long. Rajni could already feel the baby moving, they had seen him on the scan and their hearts had lifted with delight. They had been told that one operation should fix the problem – though the risk seemed very high (somehow the shocking news that the baby might or might not die at surgery had blurred into a sense of a 50:50 chance of survival – whereas in fact the chance of death was less than 5 per cent). Neither Rajni nor Ian had any real doubt; they would carry on with the pregnancy. They were warned that their baby could need a procedure to stabilize him directly after birth, even before the main operation. They had an opportunity to visit the hospital where the baby would be operated on and although they were scared by the sight of the children in intensive care, the nurses were welcoming. They met a liaison nurse who would be their contact before and after delivery. They had extra scans later in the pregnancy. Not dwelling on the future helped; both went back to work. The early diagnosis gave them the chance to tell their own parents that the grandchild they were waiting for would face a big

* This condition is called 'Transposition of the Great Arteries/Vessels', a.k.a. 'Transposition' or 'TGA' or 'dTGA' (TGV or dTGV).

challenge. With all this warning, everyone was as prepared as they could possibly be. They named the baby Jai – 'conqueror'.

Rajni went into labour a few days early. As things progressed, she and Ian sensed that a squad of people were lurking outside their hospital room, including a paediatric cardiology specialist. As Jai was born, the delivery room filled up – equipment, doctors, activity. Rajni had the briefest of cuddles before her son was taken away in an incubator and all of a sudden the room was empty; Rajni and Ian were left on their own with no baby.

They didn't see Jai again for three hours. By then the heart specialist had enlarged the natural hole between the collecting chambers to allow some mixing of the blue and red blood. It's a two-person job, done under sterile conditions: one doctor pushes a tube with a deflated balloon at its tip up from the umbilical stump towards the heart; the other person checks the balloon's progress with an ultrasound 'camera' (transducer) on the baby's abdomen or chest. The tube readily follows the course that placental blood had taken as it returned to the heart. On arriving there, it naturally falls across the hole in the atrial wall, much as Jai's blood had done before he was born. Once the tip of the tube is visible in the left atrium, the operator uses fluid to blow up the balloon on the end; on the screen you can see the balloon taking up most of the volume of the left atrium. With someone firmly holding the baby's shoulders, the balloon is then yanked backwards to tear the wall between the atria, enlarging the hole. (When teaching the technique, Bill Rashkind, who invented it in 1966, used to say, 'It's the jerk on the end that counts.') A generous hole ensures that enough red blood gets to the body to stabilize the baby for a few days before surgery is needed.

Thus the first pictures his family have of Jai were under the bright lights of a neonatal unit, festooned with tubes and looking vulnerable. Over the next days he was moved without urgency to the specialist unit where his parents met nurses they recognized, and he had the arterial switch operation that had been planned before he was born. Jai conquered each challenge and now, at the age of ten, is aiming for a black belt in tae kwon do.

Adam and Jai's problems are among a group of congenital heart conditions that make the transition to lung breathing very hazardous; they are sometimes called 'critical' congenital heart disease.* Both Adam and Jai's survival totally depended on the fetal hole between the collecting chambers persisting after birth. Others with different critical congenital heart diseases depend on the other fetal 'shortcut': the vessel outside the heart that joins the pulmonary (lung) artery to the aorta (body) artery. For some abnormal hearts, this duct is the only way into the lungs; for others the duct is the only route for blood to reach most of the body. Unfortunately for them, after birth, the very process of breathing sends a signal to the muscle in the duct wall telling it to constrict and close off the vessel. This helps in normal hearts where an open duct would make them inefficient. Unfortunately biology ensures that exactly the same process occurs in babies with heart problems; evolution has not provided a 'don't do that' switch. The process starts quickly but may take days to complete. Babies whose lung-blood supply is 'duct dependent' get gradually bluer until their low oxygen levels are unsurvivable. Babies with a 'duct-dependent' body blood supply die as lethal amounts of acid leak from the parts of the body that are not receiving enough blood.

Adam and Jai were both twenty-first-century babies. In the 1950s they would not have received the surgery they needed – newborns were not operated on until the 1960s, and even then mortality rates were still very high. This is easy to understand:

---

* Hypoplastic Left Heart Syndrome, pulmonary atresia, severe aortic or pulmonary stenosis, interrupted aortic arch and some coarctations as well as Transposition of the Great Arteries and TAPVD are conditions that make babies precarious after birth. More about some of these later.

before the late 1970s recognition, diagnosis and surgery for these babies had all to be achieved in the small time-window before the communications closed – usually just a few hours or days. A baby can collapse after birth for reasons other than heart disease and there was no quick way of checking out the heart before the development of ultrasound diagnosis. Precarious babies were reaching specialist centres day and night and being rushed into the radiology lab. Here tubes were inserted into their groins and pushed up into their hearts so that dye could be injected and diagnostic pictures taken. If surgery was feasible, perhaps for a baby with a complete block between heart and lung artery ('pulmonary atresia'), they might hurry directly to the operating room where a surgical shunt might be put in to substitute for the duct. Much of this activity would happen at night because lengthy scheduled operations would fill the operating rooms throughout the day.

After the late 1970s it was realized that the duct could be tricked into staying open. Scientists learned to synthesize prostaglandin, the hormone-like molecule that keeps the duct muscle relaxed in the fetus; it could be infused into a baby's circulation after delivery. This trick made a huge difference to the lifestyle of paediatric cardiologists and surgeons; a deteriorating baby arriving at night could be put on a prostaglandin drip, its duct would reopen and the baby would stabilize itself and be ready for diagnosis and surgery the next day. Nowadays a prostaglandin infusion is often started before the baby is transported to the specialist centre, even before a diagnosis is made.

Since the late 1980s, developments in technology and expertise have enabled reliable ultrasound diagnoses to be made before birth. This forewarning has almost certainly saved many lives, as medical staff and families have the chance to plan ahead; a prostaglandin infusion can be drawn up and ready near the delivery room, or a team can be prepared as it was for Jai. But, as Adam's story shows, critical heart defects can be missed by all the screening checks – and prostaglandins can only help if the baby actually reaches hospital care in time.

Getting deteriorating babies to hospital early enough depends on how parents or midwives act when they are worried, on how and when they call for help and on the skills of the emergency services. It is hard to say whether all these are better, worse or much the same as they were fifty years ago. Even now, a cardiac diagnosis is occasionally first made when a coroner requires a post-mortem examination on a newborn baby who unexpectedly collapsed at home.

It would be easy to attribute Adam and Jai's survival to the urgent open-heart surgery they both had soon after birth, but that story would be incomplete. But for his parent's efforts at resuscitation and the prompt arrival of a competent emergency team, Adam would probably have died on New Year's Eve. But for the eagle-eyes of the obstetric sonographer, Jai might have been born undiagnosed then crashed at home, much as Adam did. Sonographers spend most hours of most days scanning normal babies, but Jai's sonographer noticed a minimal anomaly in a tiny moving structure and acted on what she had seen. Neither the ambulance crew nor the sonographer can expect to make decisions about another baby with congenital heart disease in their whole careers, yet for Adam and Jai their responses were crucial. They are not part of the 'prestigious' specialist services that both boys relied on for the next chapter of their stories. Yet in many ways the challenges of first noticing and sorting out an unclassified problem are much greater than the predictable work of specialists who function in big teams team diagnosing and operating on arriving babies every day of the week. Perhaps the scanners and emergency services deserve as much respect.

5

'Those children are my crossword puzzles'

Mostly the rule holds true that 'being ill without a diagnosis is usually worse than being ill with one', but
Charles might be the exception where the diagnosis can be worse
than the disease. Ebstein's anomaly* causes some babies to die even
before birth, yet others, like Charles, make old bones. Though he
had been at the back of the cross-country pack at his preparatory
school, as a child he was never sickly. In his early teens, however, he
had an attack of palpitations that lasted all day (and occasioned his
unlikely bargain with God that if He would stop them, he would
never bet or gamble, except on horses). In 1960, as an optimistic
twenty-year-old medical student, Charles was admitted to Guy's
Hospital in London where a visiting Johns Hopkins team supervised the pushing of a plastic tube up from his arm to his heart; this
investigation stamped the label 'Ebstein's anomaly' on his medical
record. The announcement of most cardiac diagnoses is quickly
followed by an 'and so this is what we will do . . .' conversation,
but Ebstein's anomaly was not on the list of operable problems in
1960 and there was virtually no information about the long-term

---

* The right side of the heart, in particular the tricuspid valve, is abnormal.

outlook for people affected. Hearts preserved in pots of formalin and labelled 'Ebstein' are often kept in medical museums because the malformation looks so striking, and when Charles turned to the medical textbooks in his university library, he saw alarming pictures. He felt obliged to write a solemn letter to his girlfriend to put his cards on the table. He could not promise to live long. There were all sorts of uncertainties ahead. He was not a safe bet. She wrote back briskly and they were engaged the following week.

Charles qualified as a doctor and had a long career as an anaesthetist, though with some professional compromises. He took jobs of lower status than his first-rate training had prepared him for – 'in case' his physical capacity would let everyone down. His family came to avoid intrepid holidays 'in case' of palaver abroad. For the past thirty years he has probably never raised his pulse rate above 90, on the theory that a compromised and excitable heart needs less work and not more. He has coped with a variety of nasty rhythm problems, trying new drugs and pacemakers as they came on the market and he has needed several electric shocks to terminate attacks of palpitations. But in the fifty years since his diagnosis, life has gone on pretty well. Few friends or colleagues know that his heart is out of the ordinary and he has had no surgery. I met him when he was seventy in his beautiful rural home, happy to be a grandfather – but pensive. Looking back, it is possible that the gloom surrounding the formal *diagnosis* of an uncorrectable condition whose implications were hazy has been worse than the *disease* itself. The label suffused his subsequent life with a vague pessimism that was contrary to his nature. Who is to know if his caution has paid dividends – or undermined his potential?

★   ★   ★

For both doctor and patient, applying a fancy name to the medical problem is the usual starting point for being able to address a muddle of unanswered questions: 'What is going wrong?' 'Can anything be

done about it?' 'What does it mean for the future?' But a diagnosis
is only a name. For it to be helpful, you need a map of the territory
around it, with the possible paths to a happy future well charted
and the dangerous areas marked out. For Charles, and for many
patients diagnosed before the treatment of congenital heart disease
had evolved very far, there were few roads and no maps. Their
diagnosis only corresponded to an area marked 'Here be Dragons'.

Even now, for most doctors and nurses, the specialty of children's cardiology is akin to a foreign country whose terrain they
do not know and whose dialect they do not speak. They may
recognize that something is wrong but cannot give it a name. For
parents of newborn heart babies, news usually drips out slowly as
the anxiety of the staff around them escalates. Perhaps 'We are taking him away to give him extra oxygen,' then 'He may have a heart
problem,' then 'We need to send him to another hospital' where
'We need to do some tests' . . . right up to the crucial moment
when a specialist arrives with a diagnosis, a 'summing up'. Parents'
descriptions of these encounters convey an air of annunciation:
after hours or days of uncertainty and terrible tension, the doctor
arrives with his decisive news on which so many existential hopes
are pinned. Though they try to rally their faculties to receive his
crucial information, one parent described the experience as like
having a 'hole in your brain that information falls into when you
are not ready to receive it'. The actual name of the condition – 'the
diagnosis' – is not what they take in at the time; it is what follows
– a sketch of the consequences for their child. Usually operations
follow and, in a way they would never before have imagined, parents become 'used to this whole hospital and surgery malarkey' and
begin themselves to soak up the language of medicine.

Making a diagnosis is the archetypal activity of a physician –
corresponding to a surgeon's ability to operate. All a cardiologist's
training and technological know-how come together as they fit clues
from the patient's story, what they notice on examination and from

test results, and how and to what extent these match with a pattern seen in other people, one that authority has a name for, a name that discriminates this condition from that one. It is a completely impersonal, matter-of-fact exercise, much like solving a crossword puzzle. But for the individual born with a heart condition – the one on the receiving end – the diagnosis describes a whole existential situation, an enduring statement about himself, his present and his potential. For some people, even after treatment their heart problem will never be just incidental to their character like having blue eyes or big feet. For many, it will dominate their identity for years.

As treatments for increasingly complicated problems evolved from their beginnings in the late 1940s, diagnostic details expanded in proportion to interventions available. When nothing could be done whatever the problem, itemizing the abnormalities was not useful. In 1939, a family doctor heard a loud murmur indicating a heart problem in a newborn baby (now in his seventies) and felt under no pressure to specify what the problem was. His main responsibility was simple – to warn the parents that the baby 'might not do'. Now, an unusually jumbly heart might need twenty lines of print to describe it fully – with every detail relevant to what might happen next. The downside of the meticulous jargon that has evolved with the treatment of congenital heart disease is that, like Eskimos with many words for snow, the very complexity of the dialect used by the 'inner circle' is impenetrable even to doctors outside the specialty – and perplexing for parents who need a sympathetic interpreter. (Doctors can be like the British abroad, whose response to uncomprehending foreigners is simply to speak slowly and rather loudly in English.)*

---

* Worse, the languages used to describe complicated congenital heart diseases evolved differently on the two sides of the Atlantic. Doctors still use different terms to describe the same disease, though committees are sorting out a sort of congenital-heart-Esperanto.

It is true that doctors often identify patients by their diagnosis – 'the coarctation in the side room' – but some experienced patients also come to speak the language – 'actually I'm an Eisenmenger'. How patients talk about themselves to medical outsiders is quite another and more delicate matter. The public has no grasp of the diversity of heart problems that children can be born with. They do not know that some conditions are essentially curable while other diagnoses will take a greater toll on a childhood than having cancer. With few words available to describe heart problems, the language of stereotypes creeps in. This makes it easy for healthy people to patronize or even to demean: 'heart kid', 'blue baby', 'invalid'.

★   ★   ★

In the 1930s, 'paediatric cardiology' could not be said to exist as a specialty, yet plenty of children with heart problems were lying in hospital beds. Most had rheumatic fever, for which the main treatment was bed rest, endured for months, sometimes years. Though it would not prove to be a long-term recovery, many of these youngsters eventually got better and went home. Not so the children on the same wards with congenital heart disease – their disease would always catch up with them. Their defects had not killed them at birth but had left them debilitated by stiff lungs and breathlessness or bedridden as a result of low oxygen levels or strokes. For nurses and doctors with no hope to offer, working on these wards must have seemed a professionally dead-end job, the sort of place where an inconvenient female doctor could be sequestered away from the male-dominated mainstream.

Helen Taussig had been to university in Boston, Berkeley, Radcliffe and Harvard but none would admit a woman for a medical degree. A (female) philanthropist had bequeathed money to the Johns Hopkins Medical School in Baltimore on condition that they admit women; complying with the letter of the bequest they admitted only two each year (but only offered one a job). In

1930, Dr Taussig took up a post in the Cardiac Department of the 'Harriet Lane Home for Invalid Children', an offshoot of the Johns Hopkins Hospital. Her small team started reviewing the two hundred children (which she described as her 'crossword puzzles') for whom no detailed cardiac diagnosis had ever been made; they might have simply been labelled '*morbus caeruleus*'.* In the 1930s, their tools were simply their eyes, ears and hands. They catalogued the children's colour (very blue children have a ruddy complexion, their lips maybe the colour of a dark plum), the curvature of their chests (indicating enlargement of the heart below) and the shape of their fingertips (which take on the shape of drumsticks in blue children). They felt their necks for a buzz (technically called a 'thrill' whose position can indicate where the matching murmur originates) and noticed the flickering movements of veins in their neck (corresponding to the kick of an atrium contracting). Stethoscopes are useful for listening for gurgles in tummies or crackles in lungs but using them to discriminate between different heart murmurs is a staple part of a medical student's training. A murmur signifies turbulence somewhere underneath, perhaps from a jet of blood pumping through a hole or a narrowed valve – and it must be said that congenital heart disease offers the most exotic murmurs in the book. One patient I spoke with, Patrick, was four and understood the commercial potential of the new murmur he had acquired after his shunt operation.† When the consultant and

---

* 'Blue disease' – doctors did love their Latin. In England even in the early 1970s, a Latin qualification was a requirement for entry to medical school. The 'good' reason was that students would be better able to decode phrases like '*morbus caereleus*' but the 'real' reason was probably to keep the riff-raff out of the profession.

† This is a 'continuous murmur', blood whooshing continuously through the shunt from the high pressure (arm) vessel to the low pressure (pulmonary artery). It is quite distinctive, sometimes called a machinery murmur. A 1960s medical student would have been over the moon to add this to their tally.

his entourage arrived at his bedside he hugged his arms around his little chest, fending off the stethoscope, and demanding 'Tuppence to listen'. The consultant would sigh and put two pennies in the collection. Later the ward sister chided Pat for charging the medical students too – 'they are poor, you know' – but he was adamant; a boy needed comics and sweets.

Before the 1950s the only tests that could add information to the clinical examination would be an electrocardiogram (ECG), a blood test or an X-ray. An ECG records tiny electrical signals rippling away from the heart; they are picked up by sensors on the skin and transmitted as wiggly lines on a paper roll. The ceremony of recording an early ECG was interminable; the recording paper had to be running at just the right speed, the inky needle not too splotchy, the child was told when they could and could not breathe; twelve separate recordings had to be made and the whole process could easily take half an hour. Moreover, nobody would explain to a four-year-old that the electricity was 'coming out of' not 'going into' to their body and one woman recollects how the 'don't move' instruction terrified her because she thought she would get an electric shock.[*] (These days, once stickers are attached to the limbs and chest, an ECG recording takes only moments.)

There is no numerical scale for recording how blue a child is. One man remembers as a boy being chased upstairs by a surgeon in a pin-striped suit.[†] On each landing was a little table with a bright angle-poise light that the great man shone in his face to check the boy's colour as his oxygen levels plummeted with exercise.

---

[*] She was right to be worried. One of the 1954 cross-circulation children was electrocuted and died after surgery because the ECG machine that doctors were using to monitor his heart was not earthed properly.

[†] This was Russell, then Sir Russell, then Lord Brock. He tried standardizing blueness against a colour card like those found in paint shops, but the method did not catch on.

Most doctors resorted instead to blood tests to measure numbers of red blood cells; the lower the oxygen levels, the more red blood cells the body manufactures.* (These days, a gadget that fits on a fingertip gives a digital read-out of blood oxygen levels and can be bought over the counter in well-stocked pharmacies. Over the years, these 'pulse oximeters' must have saved blue children countless needle-sticks.)

The gee-whizz technology in doctors' offices in the 1940s was fluoroscopy, a sort of cine X-ray apparatus that had been popularized during the First World War by surgeons hunting for bullets embedded in their patient's bodies.† Dr Taussig's trainees were required each day to present what they had learned about the children on the ward to their boss and to the growing numbers of visitors. Everybody wore aviator-type goggles with red glass in them, so that when the audience shuffled in to a dim cupboard-sized fluoroscopy room, their eyes were already adapted to the dark. The bewildered child sat between a radiation source and a screen that phosphoresced when hit by the X-rays, so that spectators could see the uncanny interior of his chest and watch the lung-blood vessels dancing on the grainy screen – just like having the 'X-ray vision' of cartoons. Nobody wore a lead apron, so during the exposure both patients and viewers were receiving

---

* There are cells in the kidneys that leak a specific protein when circulating oxygen levels are low (perhaps at altitude or from an abnormal heart). The protein was isolated and named erythropoietin, now EPO. It travels through the bloodstream to the bone marrow and stimulates it to produce more red blood cells. These improve the blood's ability to carry oxygen – at the price of the extra cells sludging inside brain arteries, blocking vessels and sometimes causing strokes. This is the same EPO that has been used in blood doping in some endurance sports.

† Shoe-fitting fluoroscopes were a sales gimmick in high-end shoe stores; they allowed salesmen to check that children in the 1920s–1950s could wiggle their toes in new shoes.

doses of scattered radiation that would be far beyond the range permitted today.*

At some point after all their clinical features had been catalogued, the children usually died. Such was Dr Taussig's relationship with the parents that she would approach them to request an autopsy so that she personally could correlate her clinical findings and the patient's life story with the structural peculiarities she would see with the actual heart in her hand. Gradually distinctive patterns of clues that corresponded consistently to autopsy findings became clear and she could test her predictions in life with what the autopsy would show. After ten years of endeavour, in 1947 Dr Taussig published the first clinical textbook, *Congenital Malformations of the Heart*. The clarity that this manual brought to clinical diagnosis was a credit to Dr Taussig and her team, but the book was as much a legacy left by those doomed patients and their families for the benefit of children who might be born in a time when surgery would be possible. An eminent colleague said that the book 'brought congenital heart disease out of fairy-land' – it was the first 'map' of the territory.

This was good timing. As operations became possible for some abnormalities, a field was emerging in which, far from being an arcane 'stamp collecting' exercise, diagnosis had a serious purpose. Dr Taussig herself had come up with the idea of using the artery going to the arm to provide a second, artificial route into the lung circuit for children who were blue because of some blockage to their lung-blood flow (the 'shunt'). She presented her idea to a number of disparaging surgeons before finding her 'daring young man on the flying trapeze'. Dr Blalock and his lab technician

---

* Thyroid cancer is an unusual malignancy that is sometimes caused by radiation exposure. It may have been a coincidence, but one of Lillehei's early 1950s Fallot patients developed thyroid cancer at a young age. It was successfully treated. Medical radiation exposure is much more tightly regulated now.

Vivien Thomas already knew, having experimented on dogs for a different purpose, that vessels heading towards the arms could be located as they left the chest, then cut and successfully plumbed into the lung artery. For the child with a low lung-blood flow, the surgical 'shunt' would simply pipe blood continuously from the high-pressure (arm) to the low-pressure (lung) vessel. The first human 'Blalock-Taussig shunt' was performed at the Johns Hopkins Hospital in late November 1944. By October 1950, the team in Baltimore had undertaken 1,000 shunt operations. In the early days of publicity, the clinic was receiving over 100 letters and telegrams every week and parents were turning up unbooked at the hospital, hoping for an operation for their child. The diagnostic problem then facing Dr Taussig was sorting those who might benefit from a shunt from those who would not.

All the arrivals were blue and it's a fair bet that, like Dick Ket, most had Fallot's tetralogy. Even in 1888, Fallot himself said (in French) 'cyanosis, especially in the adult, is the result of a small number of well-determined cardiac malformations. One is much more frequent than the others (*the tetralogy*); this is what the clinician should diagnose and in doing so his chances of error are relatively slight.' Guessing and being wrong mattered little to docteur Fallot – he could do nothing for his patients anyway; but for Dr Taussig, guessing and being wrong meant sending the wrong child to surgery, and this would probably mean their death.

Although the surgeon did need to open the chest to create the shunt, there was no need to open up the heart itself, so it was not necessary to be too accurate about what was going on inside it. But Dr Taussig *did* have to prevent any children whose 'plumbing' made them blue for a completely different reason going to surgery. Some very blue children might already have perfectly adequate blood flows to their lungs, but a defect that made the streaming of blue and red blood inside the heart hopelessly wrong

– children like Jai in the previous chapter, whose parents were told even before he was born that his aorta came off his right ventricle and his pulmonary artery off his left ventricle (Transposition of the Great Arteries). Or children born with a Ventricular Septal Defect (VSD) might arrive looking blue because their lung-blood vessels had already been ravaged by high blood flows earlier in life and the tipping point reached when blue blood returning from the body was finding it easier to cross 'right to left' across the VSD and go out to the body – the Eisenmenger situation that Madhubala was in when she died. A shunt would be the last thing that a child with either Transposition or Eisenmenger needed. Some arrivals were indeed turned away, including a mother who had hitchhiked from West Virginia to Baltimore carrying her very blue child in the hope of help.

Unfortunately, the diagnostic process so carefully documented by Dr Taussig in her book was still fallible. In the days before the internet and the conference-travel industry, surgical publications were more extensive and mistakes were much better documented than is usual today. Reporting his first fifty-seven operations to the world, Blalock mentioned shunting a patient with Eisenmenger's syndrome and another with Transposition of the Great Arteries and that both children had died. What Dr Taussig really needed was some safe, non-surgical means to get inside these abnormal hearts to track the paths of the blue and red blood and measure pressures in the heart's chambers, but these techniques were still some years away.

Mistaken diagnosis was a major problem in the early days of open-heart surgery too. In the early 1950s, it was a lot harder to find a cardiologist competent to diagnose what was wrong with a child's heart than to find a surgeon keen to operate inside it. In their enthusiasm to be in the forefront of their field, they were over-confident in a diagnostic process that was not up to the job of correctly predicting what they would find once they were

inside a heart; as a result, there were a series of disasters leading
to patients' deaths on the operating table. In April 1951, thinking
they would find an Atrial Septal Defect (ASD), surgeons chose a
five-year-old girl called Patty Anderson for the 'first in-human'
outing for a prototype machine that could take over the work of
her heart for the five minutes they anticipated that closing the
hole would take. She died on the operating table. The heart–lung
machine that they had been carefully testing had functioned, but
the diagnosis had been wrong.* In February 1952, a different
surgeon anticipated closing an ASD using a different prototype
machine and his patient also died on the operating table, with
blood overflowing the open chest and spilling on to the floor –
another incorrect diagnosis.† In a report from England in 1953,
the main problem documented among the first 200 shunt operations at Guy's Hospital in London was that the surgeon could
not even find a pulmonary artery on to which to put a shunt.
There had been too much guessing and 'hoping for the best';
cardiologists needed to raise their game.

To avoid these diagnostic errors, doctors needed to be able to
actually check the pressures and blood flows in the chambers of
a child's heart – and ideally obtain some more detailed pictures.
Research scientists had pushed flexible tubes around the circulations of animals, but people (including patients) worried that the
human heart might stop if it was poked from within. The first
to push a tube into a human heart was a German medical intern

* The surgeon was Clarence Dennis working in Minneapolis. In fact, Patty did
not have a straightforward ASD but the much more complicated lesion that we
now call an Atrioventricular Septal Defect.
† This was Dr Gibbon working in Philadelphia. The child did not have an atrial
hole at all but a ductus, which could have been fixed without even opening
her heart.

in 1929, operating on himself.* Gradually through the 1930s and 1940s, a few doctors on both sides of the Atlantic drove forward this technology. They established that touching the heart was safer than anticipated and that it was practical to measure pressures inside the circulation and even take blood samples. By 1947, a team in the Harvard Medical School had wiggled tubes up into and through the right side of the heart and on out into the lung artery and had measured the pressures and oxygen levels in the hearts of adults.

By the mid 1950s, cardiologists had started pushing flexible tubes around children's hearts to better establish what was going on inside them. This could be an ordeal of a completely different order from anything Dr Taussig's team had imposed on her early patients. With no parent in the vicinity and often while wide awake, a young child would be settled on a hard table, surrounded by huge and unfamiliar mechanical equipment, with gowned and masked figures looming over them in the near-pitch-dark. Local anaesthetics numbed their arms or groins before the cardiologist would cut through their skin to find a vein big enough to take a catheter-tube. These tests might last two or three hours. When,

---

* This was Werner Forssmann. The story goes that his proposal to try the procedure on himself was vetoed by his boss but he persuaded an operating theatre nurse to help him with his plan. She agreed on condition that *she* was the volunteer. He strapped her onto an operating table and injected some local anesthetic into her skin – and also surreptitiously his own. Then he exposed a vein in his own elbow and threaded a tube into his own vein, talking to Gerda all the while. By the time she realized she had been tricked, a long length of tube had run up Forssmann's arm and she was released from the restraints and escorted Werner upstairs to the X-ray department where fluoroscopy showed the catheter obviously in his heart. German bosses dislike disobedience and the stunt was bad for Forssmann's career – and the Second World War even worse. When in 1956 he shared a Nobel prize in Medicine he was the go-to doctor for prostatic gentlemen in a German spa town.

over sixty years later, I asked about their childhood catheterization tests from the 1950s, several people had very lucid recollections, others had 'flashback' images. Children may have been given some sleepy medicines that may have altered their understanding of what was going on, but we have no choice about the childhood memories we carry with us over decades.

Mary Jane just relived her misery; she had cried completely unconsoled throughout the procedure. Diana had absolutely no memory of the test itself, but remembered waking up mystified by little black stitches that seemed to have 'grown' in her arm. Judith remembers the alarming all-over-flush and the sensation that her head would blow off (as dye passed around her circulation) leaving her feeling as though she had wet herself. Marilyn recalled the weird scratching inside her body as the catheter tube was pushed towards her heart; once she had to climb off the table onto a gurney in order to be moved from one hospital to another, tube in situ. Rita had been treated in Boston in 1954 and remembers feeling completely fearless; the evening before the test a 'beautiful' nurse had explained what was to happen. Aged seven, she had her right arm stretched out and tied down. They tilted her head to the left and put a cloth over the side of her face. The doctors sported shiny aprons and goggles similar to those worn by divers. When the lights went out, nursery figures were being projected on to the ceiling, but she was more interested in watching the reflection of the X-ray screen in the doctors' goggles. In the same era in London, nobody had thought to warn five-year-old Coralie about the test. Lying motionless and disregarded in the pitch-dark during her catheterization through her groin, she had a definite thought: 'those men shouldn't be touching me down there'. Many years later when she was training as a psychotherapist, she addressed this memory and realized that she had carried throughout childhood a sort of uncertainty that she might have been sexually abused in some way that day.

All these patchy memories are completely plausible, including the moving from one hospital to another. To obtain an image of the heart, a doctor would inject some radiopaque dye and quickly take some X-rays as it whooshed through the cardiac chambers and out. In those days, putting dyes into the body was the province of radiologists, not cardiologists, and the two sorts of doctor might even work in different hospitals, or on different days of the week. To avoid a child having two procedures, in Great Ormond Street Hospital in the 1950s the cardiologist would put the catheter tube in and measure pressures and oxygen levels. He would then position the catheter tip where he wanted the dye to be injected, strap the tube to the child's leg and move the patient six floors down in a rickety lift, along some very public corridors and into the basement of another building were the radiologist would take over to inject the dye and record the pictures (angiograms). When the dye had been squirted in, a technician slid photographic plates manually, one at a time, into a unit under the table that the child was lying on. With blood leaving the heart at about three feet per second, he had to be slick to catch even one decent image of the heart as the bolus of radiopaque dye passed through the heart. Then the photographic plates would take four hours to develop, so the child would be awake and back in the ward before anyone knew if the dye had even been injected into the right place.

In the early days, doctors did not devote much attention to what we now call the 'patient experience'; for example, a medical demarcation dispute might mean that a child had two unpleasant experiences – a catheterization and an angiogram – in two days. But all the doctors wanted to learn: Marilyn had ten catheterizations before she was seventeen, all without sedation, and I suspect that many of these were more for the trainee doctors' benefit than for Marilyn's. With time, the process became more civilized: cutting the skin to get access to veins became unnecessary, the radiologists agreed that cardiologists could inject dyes, the technology became less clunky, sedation regimes or full anaesthesia became the norm for children and the doctors' facility at 'driving' their tubes around complex circulations improved vastly. But by the time cardiac catheterization and angiography had become more humane, it was going out of fashion for making a diagnosis.

In truth, catheterization and angiography never did solve all possible diagnostic problems; for instance they are not good at visualizing the valves inside the heart. In the early 1980s, and despite more than one angiogram, details of the interior of James's heart remained a bit of a mystery. He seemed to have two pumping chambers but a huge hole between them. The normal heart has four valves that maintain the one-way flow of blood; they are flimsy flaps of tissue that open and shut like doors. The tricuspid valve – the 'trapdoor' in the floor of the right atrium – slams shut under pressure when the right ventricle squeezes blood out towards the lungs and opens again when the ventricle relaxes. The valve/'closed door' protects the atrium and veins behind the door from the pressure surge. The valve/door is tethered by cords like 'guy-ropes' that prevent it flipping upwards and causing a leak. The 'tent pegs' of the cords are anchored in the muscle of the ventricle and in James's heart there was concern that they were fastened into the left (wrong) ventricle. If this were true, closing the hole in his heart would wreck the 'guy ropes' and stop his tricuspid valve from working properly. Making a decision about which would be the best (or least worst) operation for James hinged on establishing if it would be safe to close the hole – and no angiogram would sort this out. So when a new piece of kit – the two-dimensional (2D) echo machine – was first bought by his hospital, James was invited down to see if the latest technology would solve the problem. Thin, fast-moving valves were just the sort of thing that the 2D echo was good at imaging.

In the late 1970s, news that a machine was being test-driven spread through the hospital where I was training. I remember queuing to enter a darkened room where my ecstatic boss was riveted by a tiny screen showing a green blob flipping in and out of the left ventricle with the heartbeat. This was a rare cardiac tumour swinging around precariously on a stalk. To have a diagnosis of 'left atrial myxoma' confirmed was shocking for the patient, but for the spectators it was party time – a view into the future of cardiac diagnosis. The days of diagnosis being an esoteric pattern-recognition exercise using clues from examination, tests and fleeting shadows of a heart outlined by dye were over. With 2D echo imaging, diagnosis became something that you could point to – 'there's the problem'.

'Ultra' sound, in the sense of sound inaudible to humans, was first generated artificially in the late nineteenth century and by the First World War, SOund Navigation And Ranging (SONAR) was being used to detect submarines. By the late 1940s, there was a lot of experience with bouncing ultrasound waves off underwater objects to measure their depth, but nobody had tried to use the technology to work on the much smaller scale of the human body. In Sweden in 1953, fate brought together the director of a catheterization lab (Dr Inge Edler) and a boy-wonder physics student (the not-yet-Dr Hertz).* At the time, the only commercial use of short-distance ultrasound was in testing for industrial metal fatigue, so Hertz visited a shipyard and played with their weld-testing kit. When he put their 'reflectoscope' on his own chest he noticed a signal corresponding to his heartbeat coming back onto the screen and borrowed the equipment for the weekend to show his collaborator. They could not raise money to buy an instrument to experiment with, but Hertz's eminent dad had connections. So while on his honeymoon in Germany, Helmuth

---

* Helmuth Hertz came from a famous physics family: his father was Gustave Hertz, Nobel Prizewinner and his uncle Heinrich Hertz, who gave his name to the unit of sound frequency.

Hertz excused himself from his new wife to visit the Siemens factory where industrial ultrasound 'reflectoscopes' were being built. When Hertz showed the developers his trick of picking up reflections from the human heart, the Siemens commercial team immediately recognized the potential of the technology. Hertz went off with a machine on long-term loan and the whole field of medical ultrasound scanning was born.

The first machines could only gauge the distance from the 'camera'/transducer on the chest wall to the structure off which the ultrasound waves bounced, and in 1953 the first photographic recordings were underwhelming. Edler had to go to a lot of trouble to prove what the signals corresponded to. He carried out ultrasound examinations on dying patients: with the transducer on their chests, he found the pulsatile signal and carefully marked the point where the transducer touched their skin and the exact direction of the beam. Then, after the patient died, in a 'Scandinavian noir' gesture, he put an ice pick on the spot on the cadaver's chest and pushed it in the beam's direction; the ice pick penetrated the muscle of the right (front) ventricle, passed through the wall between the chambers and out through the back of the heart, proving the source of the signal. Using the same equipment, his local obstetrical colleague produced the first ultrasound diagnosis of twins in utero, but the tool did not seem to offer much to cardiologists and the impetus to develop ultrasound in cardiology fizzled out in Sweden.

The next phase of development was not until the 1970s and was largely in the USA. The generation of the sort of 2D pictures of the heart that we see today depended on coupling the ultrasound beam to the same sort of mechanism that makes the whirr of an electric toothbrush. Coming when it did, echo technology had great 'purchase' in terms of improving anatomical understanding of children's hearts and it remains the mainstay of real-life diagnosis today. The discomfort and hazards of cardiac catheterization could often be avoided. The echo pictures of the 1980s were still fuzzy by present standards and when James's parents were asked to formally consent to his surgery, they signed their permission for any one of three possible operations, depending on whether or not the difficulties with his tricuspid valve were confirmed.

Echo technology continued to evolve. Patients now describe the images as 'like science fiction'; jets of blood travelling at high velocity can be 'seen' in colour. The camera-probes usually pressed on to the chest can also be sited in the oesophagus behind the heart (allowing surgical results to be checked on the operating table) or in the vagina (to look at very early pregnancies.) Computer techniques can reconstruct a 3D image from a sweep of 2D scans – 'incredible'.

Competing in terms of amazing pictures is Magnetic Resonance Imaging (MRI) technology. Though the patient will be more aware of the noise and claustrophobia than the physics, a *magnetic* field is applied to them and all the protons in all the water molecules in their body align and begin to spin together (*resonate*). When the magnet is turned off, each proton gives up a little energy as it goes back to its less ordered configuration; the energy released takes the form of a radio wave that is picked up and processed by a computer directed from a sort of 'mission control' room adjacent to the scanner. This turns the radio signals into a 2D *image* or 'slice'. Slices stacked up can be used to construct 3D images of extraordinary detail and if trouble is taken to synchronize the magnet action with the heart's motion, a moving image can be generated.

MRI scans involve no radiation, no needles, nobody even touches your body – but scans can undoubtedly be an ordeal. The problem is that the magnets are housed around a sort of tunnel into which the patient slides and is left alone with his or her thoughts. The magnets are powerful enough to suck metal objects into the tunnel from a distance,* so everyone entering the room is frisked.

---

* The internet offers photos of metal chairs, industrial cleaners, guns and oxygen cylinders that have been inadvertently sucked into MRI magnet-tunnels.

Amelia was twenty-five years old before her heart condition was diagnosed. The basic problem was evident from examining her, and looking at her ECG and cardiac echo, she had sub-aortic stenosis, a progressive blockage within her left ventricle underneath her aortic valve. An MRI scan would show if her aortic valve would need replacing as part of any surgery. She was a level-headed young woman, a graduate who had been around the world with her boy-friend, but she was new to hospitals. On the day of the MRI, she chivvied family away, expecting to cope on her own.

Those who have donned a hospital gown know that – whatever the intention – they render all free spirits submissive to the regime. Although Amelia already knew she would need an operation, chan-ging into a blue robe felt serious; suddenly she understood 'I'm a patient'. In the changing room she took a selfie and sent the picture to her boyfriend. Metal-free, she progressed into the MRI room and lay on the table. She felt unpleasantly pinioned by the anti-wriggle board that was put over her, trapped and helpless. As the table slid into the tunnel she was embarrassed to let out an involuntary little scream; she had never thought of herself as claustrophobic. It took a second attempt to settle her in the tun-nel. Then the noise. Alone in this weird situation, she struggled resolutely with her rising panic; it was calming sometimes to be told when to hold her breath. Somehow all the fears that had been brewing echoed around in this confined space, though towards the end of forty-five minutes she had hit some sort of meditative stride. But she was enormously relieved to get out.

The 'old school' examination skills on which Helen Taussig relied are not quite lost, but for the new breed of cardiologist, bedside diagnosis has surrendered utterly to the taking of high-tech pictures. With the diagnosis of complex congenital heart disease no longer the 'crossword puzzle' challenge that it once was, a trainee using current imaging techniques can make all but the most esoteric diagnosis after a year's apprenticeship. What then does a specialist offer that a trainee could not? The specialist's job is to oversee the whole range of congenital heart disease, from the most straightforward tiny hole that will close on its own, to the unique heart that will never be completely repaired. A specialist is familiar with the map of the whole territory. Given a particular diagnosis in a particular child, there are now many possible routes for getting from A to B, and an experienced doctor will understand the pros and cons of all the options. A very experienced one will also consider the option of staying where you are.

Since the 1940s, less has changed for parents, and their initial shock at hearing the diagnosis has probably barely altered. It is as though they arrive as bewildered refugees in a foreign country whose language they do not speak – and the diagnostic label that the specialist gives to their child assigns them to live in a small town with an unfamiliar name. They do not know if the diagnosis corresponds to a tranquil spot or if is in the middle of a war-zone; in time they come to know this neighbourhood only too well.

Unlike parents, specialists have a very nuanced sense of the ranking of severity within the range of congenital heart diseases; they would grade Hypoplastic Left Heart as more severe than Fallot's tetralogy, which is in turn worse than ASD. Parents don't have this perspective – why should they? If you ask them which sort of heart problem is the worst, their answer must surely be 'The one my child has.'

6
When did you last see a blue baby?

In the early days, when children had to be visibly handicapped by blueness or fatigue before a surgeon could justify the risk of a major operation, their difficulties would be obvious to us as we saw them out in the street or at school. But now that surgical confidence has increased, many children born with the same defects as those original patients have had their operations before they learn to walk and we never see them struggling. Dick Ket, the Dutch artist, and Mickey Shaw, the cross-circulation survivor, both had Fallot's tetralogy, and before 1980 many of the blue children seen getting around as best they could had the same condition; but by 2013, three-quarters of Fallot repairs performed in the UK were carried out before the child's first birthday. Only one of those 340 children died at operation and the rest were already pink by the time they were learning to walk; Fallot is now thought of as quite a favourable diagnosis.

Without the occasional reminder of catching sight of a 'blue baby', many people are mystified by the notion that there are modern 'heart children' for whom every day is still a bit of a battle. Though the unpractised eye will rarely notice them, barely-blue children are still in our midst. They are kids with a new sort of difficulty. Most were born with a problem for which surgery simply had nothing to offer before the 1980s; their predecessors with the same conditions would die very young. Many have hearts that cannot be corrected in the sense of building a normal circulation – for instance hearts that have only one useful pumping chamber. What surgery currently proposes for them is a series of operations during childhood – 'stage 1', 'stage 2', 'stage 3' – designed to eventually leave their circulations as effective as possible in order to give them a decent quality and length of life. Because the operations can only offer a 'second best' circulation, these children are easily tired and many are a bit blue. Are these children's lives at home and at school so different from those of the 'blue babies' born before 1980? And what about the impact of these children's fickle health on their mothers' plans for their own lives?

Several decades separated their childhoods from the thoughtful conversations I had with survivors of early operations – and with some of their parents; though now elderly, they had no difficulty in remembering the atmosphere of apprehension that had surrounded their child's early years. For all their experiences of doctors, hospitals and surgery, most heart children of any era spend most of their childhood at home. There, to paraphrase Tolstoy, 'each coping family copes its own way'.

Born in 1961 in New Jersey, Mary Jane's parents did not 'baby' her, and with seven siblings she was not always the centre of attention. All the children had chores. Mary Jane was always given the 'quiet' jobs, perhaps folding clothes, while siblings took out the trash, vacuumed or shovelled snow. Her parents allowed her to try physical things like playing baseball or riding a bike, though they might stand nearby quietly praying that she wouldn't drop dead. Their parenting style meant that Mary Jane did not have much insight into her 'difference' until the age of seven when she visited the girl next door and matter-of-factly asked her 'How bad are your chest pains today?' She went home to report her friend's staggering comment to her mother; the explanations and prayers that followed proved a turning point, the beginning of a real understanding that she was 'special' and why.

In England, Muriel was widowed in the mid 1960s. At around the same time, the doctors confirmed that her two-year-old daughter's frailty related to a serious heart condition. Over the next few years, her little girl spent a lot of time in bed – partly because that was the 'done thing'* but also because their home had no central heating. Muriel was a schoolteacher and, as a single parent, needed to work. Friends and neighbours could be organized to babysit, but if her daughter was sent home unexpectedly from nursery, cover was impossible to arrange (no mobile phones) and Muriel would sometimes have to leave her poorly four-year-old alone in the house, only dropping in to check on her during her lunch-break. There was no daytime television; no computer games, no audiobooks, no videos, and no library books to help pass the time. That daughter is now a mother herself and can hardly comprehend how exhausted, stretched and anxious her own mother must been.

As we talked, stories of separateness often cropped up in the reminiscences of early patients. This flashback is one of Muriel's daughter's earliest memories. She was looking wistfully out of an upstairs window watching her sister and the other kids playing in the street below; they were laughing and each had a bag of crisps.

---

* In 1947, a questioner of received truths called Dr Richard Asher provoked his colleagues by writing a paper called 'The Dangers of Going to Bed'. In those days, bed-rest was an important part of the prescription for many illnesses and the medical establishment took Asher's comments as criticism. It took them another twenty years to catch up with the statement's truth. Recounting how Asher was ostracized, his obituary explained: 'Iconoclasm was ill received in medicine's marble halls and eccentricity was only acceptable after a dedicated climb up the conformist ladder.'

This little girl already knew that she was missing out, and she was only three years old. In all the nostalgic conversations I had with patients about our common 1950s and 1960s childhoods, this was the image that conjures up the isolation, even claustrophobia, of a child who can't get out to enjoy the delight of being away from watchful parental eyes.

For we were a generation of children that played in the street, but in the 1950s and 1960s a breathless child couldn't get out under their own steam. The now-familiar collapsible strollers or baby buggies were not sold until 1969. A child who was unable to walk far depended on others if they were ever to venture outside. James, now in his sixties, told me how he used to climb on his big brother's back and beg him to carry him across the fields to play in the disused coal pits. Later his parents bought a three-wheel trike; he did not have the puff to ride it himself, but if someone was prepared to put a rope around the handlebars and pull, he could go anywhere. Marilyn remembers how her friends would cross their hands to make a seat as she draped her arms over their shoulders to carry her home. Judith only got out of the house on warm weekends, when her father would push her in a wheelchair to the shops where the nice grocer at Victor Values would give her an apple. Boys and their dads seemed to do a lot of train-watching. Not everyone was lucky; when he first went into hospital for surgery at the age of four, Patrick was so blue and breathless that he had not yet learned to walk. His family was shambolic, with a backdrop of grim inner-city poverty and casual violence. His mother was perpetually contending with pregnancies and infants and a controlling man, so nobody was taking Pat out for walks. Going into hospital was to be a revelation.

When I asked Nick, an adamantly uncomplaining man, about the loneliness of being an only child who could rarely get out, he admitted it had been tough. As a young child stranded at home, he listened to the radio soaps aimed at housewives – *Mrs Dale's*

*Diary, The Archers** – and most of his 'friends' were adults. He had indulgent neighbours and his father would take him down to look at the Altrincham Fire Station where his hero was a fireman who would sometimes let him sit on the leather seat of the fire engine; he had been heartbroken when the man moved away.

Siblings at least bring some youthful life into the house, but then as now they can have a tough time. When Rita was born in 1947 with pulmonary stenosis and Atrial Septal Defect (ASD),† her Rhode Island parents were told that she would not live very long and she now understands that her little sister was probably conceived to replace her. The household rule was that if Rita couldn't do something, her sister couldn't either – so no tap-dance lessons. But it didn't work the other way around – if Rita got presents when she came home from hospital, it did not mean that her sister would too. Yet Rita doesn't remember any moaning. For all the disappointments they endured, it's easy to believe that many siblings who have needed to learn life's lessons at a young age will mature into especially decent human beings.

Arguably, for the heart children themselves, life at home has looked up over the years, particularly for those with low energy

---

* Other British children remembered *Listen with Mother* when the BBC launched daytime television and some US patients of that era recalled listening to the Lone Ranger on the radio. (Nick may be interested to learn that Elizabeth Pargetter (née Archer) was born a little after him with the same congenital heart condition.)

† Pulmonary stenosis and ASD. The pulmonary valve is stiff and blocks the way out from right ventricle to the lungs. Blood backs up behind the obstruction and some blue blood arriving in the right atrium takes the path of least resistance and 'shunts' into the left side of the heart and is pumped around the body. Rita's whole life has been overshadowed by this problem – which is now easily tackled with a balloon passed through a vein and blown up to un-bung the valve. She reproached me for asking if she felt bitter that this quick and easy treatment had not been available for her: 'How could you not feel happy for children now?'

levels. Now, there are all sorts of screens to entertain children who are laid up on a sofa and, even if their stamina is poor, youngsters can be strapped into a buggy and trundled to the shops or the park to be part of a family outing. But if Mary Jane, James, Marilyn, Pat, Nick or Rita had been born twenty years later, they and their families would have been spared most of the experiences they described because one of the most noticeable trends in surgery for congenital heart disease over the past fifty years is the move to operating earlier and earlier in life.

In that interval, many other things have also changed affecting family life. In 1951, when cardiac surgery for children was beginning, UK and US census data showed that only one in six of mothers of young children worked outside the home; currently it is almost seven out of ten in both the UK and USA. These days, if someone has to stay at home to look after a precarious child, possibly for months or years, it is usually the mother – and the father may need to spend all possible time at work to maintain the family income. Grandparents may live miles away, neighbours are often out at work and a child-minder who will take on a poorly child is hard to find – and for most families, money is too tight for such extra expenditure.

In the 'new millennium', Gill was a competent professional woman and in 2004 was living in Scotland, pregnant with her second child and planning to move into a bigger house in Edinburgh to accommodate the larger family. Late in her pregnancy a scan showed the left side of the baby's heart to be so small as to be of little use, a situation that would not be sustainable after birth without an operation. Had Michael been born twenty years earlier when hospitals had nothing to offer it is unlikely that he would have survived, even for a week. But the baby's delivery was managed so that resuscitation expertise was ready. Wearing infant-sized ear-defenders (which the family has kept), the baby travelled 300 miles in an RAF Sea-King helicopter from Lossiemouth to

Birmingham, England, supervised by four burly uniformed attend-
ants and two lovely paramedic nurses. His 'stage 1' and 'stage 2'
operations and their aftermaths took up much of the first year of his
life; during those months his family often felt that their baby actually belonged to the hospitals and they were simply borrowing him
sometimes. Gill had all the legal entitlements to maternity leave that
the UK welfare state mandates, but soon after she struggled back
to work she was sacked. Without two secure incomes, the family
had to downsize; they moved out of town and Gill began to work
from home. Her son is now through 'stage 3' but still attached to
hospital apron strings. Like so many parents, Gill and her husband
have made one compromise after another as they got on with the
project of raising a 'different' child. But on reflection, they concede
that supporting their child may have given the whole family a sanity
and sense of proportion that they would not otherwise have had.

   Not all superheroes wear capes; I feel for all the mothers.
Muriel's present-day successors, whose daughters have conditions
that we now think of as tractable problems, have an easier time.
Bringing straightforward surgery forward into babyhood averts
years of having to adapt to setbacks. But Gill and her contemporaries whose children have more complex diagnoses still put
their own needs aside in order to offer their children the chance
of making the best of their compromised lives. Those mothers'
ways of life diverge from the lifestyles of the friends they grew up
with who have given birth to more 'ordinary' children. Mothers
in Gill's situation are less free to go out to work than their own
mothers had been and, if their children are 'frequent-fliers' to our
present-day hospitals, I sense that their tough script has become
lonelier over time.

   Gill's son is typical of the children now alive thanks to an oner-
ous series of operations that build what his support group sweetly
call a 'man-made heart'. Unlike their contemporaries, entering
school is not their first big hurdle in life, but they will have to

deal with questions about their scars and may not run about quite as energetically as their classmates. 'Purple gills', 'scar chest', 'eating blackjacks',* 'the purple', 'worm hole'. Name-calling and nicknames are a commonplace part of everyone's childhood, but when pressed, some middle-aged survivors let drop recollections of how painful those names felt. Especially before doctors even talked to children directly, a five- or six-year-old went to school with no vocabulary to explain their singularity to themselves, let alone to others. Saying that you have a 'weak heart' does not close down any teasing that happens as five-year-olds size each other up and jostle themselves into clusters of allies. To have been small and blue and a bit of a loner at school was a common experience for 'unrepaired' heart children before 1980 – and quite likely for some less-than-corrected children now. Of course, heart children do not have the monopoly of victimization, and not all heart children experience it or are necessarily very upset by it. One woman credits her three older siblings as her 'playground protectors', another attributes her escape to her own spiky attitude and a third to the teacher's matter-of-fact announcement on the very first day of his first term that he had a heart problem and deserved particular respect.†

Looking different, missing a lot of school and not keeping up in the playground served to underline in some young minds that there was something fundamentally 'wrong' with what they *were*. Guilt is a discomfort about something we *do* and it may have some useful purpose as we learn to think about other people's feelings. But it is hard to see that shame about what we *are* has any corresponding

---

* A retro liquorice-flavoured sweet that coloured your tongue and lips black.
† Teachers' announcements were not always so reliable. Geoffrey was well known in the school for being blue and needing a runner when he was batting at cricket. When he was heading off to London for his big operation, the headmaster announced in assembly that Geoffrey would be away for a while to have his blood changed.

benefit. One lass had undergone some surgery, but was still frail and needed to wear a hat and gloves outside in cold weather. A girly gang would chase her around the playground hoping she would collapse. When they shoved her hat and gloves down the toilet, she told nobody – not her teacher, not her parents. Looking back from middle age, her memory is of an intense humiliation about being different, a shame that she took upon herself.* For many early children, a transformative operation often happened at some stage; their colour and their energy levels improved and all of a sudden they could pass for 'normal'. But as adults looking back, childhood nicknames serve as a sort of enduring avatar of what they had been. It's a safe bet that the ugly duckling who felt exiled, 'ashamed to show his face, afraid of what others might say', did not forget his nickname, even after he looked at himself in the lake and saw that he had transformed over the wintertime to become a 'very fine swan indeed'.†

Bullying that tapped into real fear was, of course, the worst sort. James's heart would never be normal, though he had had some palliative surgery. In the late 1980s he was blue and breathless, a very frustrated little boy. At his worst, he was too tired to walk across a room – he might simply sink into sleep. After his class of seven-year-olds was told about the 'big op' he was facing, two boys ran around the playground calling out 'James is going to die, James is going to die!' He was terribly upset. His mother came to fetch him, the school did some damage limitation and when he next attended, everyone was particularly sweet. Twenty years later, as they described that low point of James's rollercoaster life-story,

---

* Alice Munro said: 'You cannot let your parents anywhere near your real humiliations.'
† *The Ugly Duckling* is a film, based on a Hans Christian Andersen folktale, in which Danny Kaye sings a song about a cygnet who is bullied for being 'an ugly duckling' but who then, over winter, turns into a swan.

mother and son looked knowingly at each other – those boys could have been right.

When pre-1980s children actually got to school, their education was not necessarily straightforward. If a child was very blue, its brain was 'running on empty'. Anyone who has been to an altitude above about 10,000 feet will tell you they initially felt pretty rotten – it has been described as walking on a treadmill while breathing through a straw. The doctor for the 1924 Everest expedition reported that at Base Camp (17,500 feet): 'Though the mind was clear, yet there was a disinclination for effort. It was far more pleasant to sit about than to do a job of work that required thought . . . Though mental work is a burden at high altitudes, yet with an effort it can be done.' This description chimes so well with Guy's portrayal of his primary schooling in the late 1970s. 'Teachers came to ignore me when I drifted off in school-time into the fields, daydreaming. In retrospect it was a fight just to keep going. It was hard to walk in a straight line on the flat, or even to read aloud.' But the fuzziness was reversible. One man well remembers waking clear-headed from his major operation at the age of thirteen, and realizing that he had lived his earlier life 'in a bit of a blur'. Without knowing much about blood and oxygen levels, many of the early blue children spent years with their brains working at degrees of oxygen deprivation at which pilots are obliged to wear oxygen masks.*

Time off school for illness or operations – or school phobia – gradually impact on any child's education, making it easy to

---

* Aeroplane cabins are pressurised to oxygen availability equivalent to the levels at about 8,000 feet; the dreaded oxygen masks are deployed if an emergency causes cabin decompression to 10,000 feet level equivalents. Aviation regulations require pilots to be breathing oxygen above 14,000 feet equivalents. The body can acclimatize to some extent to chronic low oxygen saturations but testing easily shows some deficits in brain function at these altitudes. (Oxygen masks would not have helped the blue children, most of whose lack of blood oxygen related to low lung-blood flows.)

understand that keeping up academically in ordinary schools is not easy for any child who often misses lessons. Repeating years and 'remedial classes' along with children who were 'a little bit different' was the 'solution' that some primary schools offered. But during the 1950s and 1960s in England, it was common for 'disabled' children to be educated separately. These 'special schools' were sometimes residential, and were often referred to as 'schools for spastics', though some had more upbeat names like 'open air schools'. There, children needing callipers for polio, wheelchairs for cerebral palsy or supervision for epilepsy were educated together – a real mix of physical and intellectual difficulties. Children with heart disease who were very limited, usually by blueness, were often channelled to these places, both before and after surgery.

Bernhard travelled to his 'special school' by taxi at the local authority's expense. There, children were arranged on benches with those further up the bench being the higher achievers; with a lot of effort, he eventually managed to get into the top half of the bench. At lunchtime, everyone rested on a bed with their name on it – if Bernhard fainted in class, that was where he would wake up. He was very happy there, the environment was caring, but by his teenage years and despite some surgery he had lost three or four years of schooling and when he left at the age of sixteen he had never taken an exam. Worse, his schooling had sheltered him from able-bodied children and the messy breadth of human behaviour, so when he ventured into the 'big wide world' he was unprepared. By then he was pink and his scars were under his shirt. Things were expected of him of which he had no real understanding. Now in his sixties, Bernhard remembers being scared – confused about signals that he was not picking up. Brought up with an expectation that people always did the right thing, every violation needed to be understood. He found it hard know what to believe or to gauge whom to trust, and some people exploited his gullibility: a 'friend' wanted to borrow money, a boss tried to avoid paying compensation for an accident at work. He was presentable and popular with the girls but relationships had not been part of his education, let alone sex. When a girl took him back to her bedroom, he sat on the bed not knowing what to do, not even knowing what he did not know. Work, friendships, brothers all gradually put him straight, but physicality came late to his relationship with his future wife; the massive scars on his chest were never mentioned. The couple are still together.

Susan's first school was the Franklin D. Roosevelt School for Physically Disabled Children, in London – overlooking the John Keats School for Delicate Children, whose pupils were envied because they got to sit out on a balcony. Again, the school environment was very caring, with a structured day and a sleep in the afternoon. The school had a choir, but education was very basic – she remembers a lot of basket-weaving. She was very happy but left barely able to read, so that when presented with the 11+ examination – which allocated children to secondary school according to their ability – she had no real grasp even of the questions being asked. Much later and a teacher herself, Susan can only suppose that she was being beautifully cared for but not educated, on the presumption that she was going to die very young. This is certainly what her parents believed.

★ ★ ★

The death rate for childhood heart surgery plummeted in the years before 2000, and since then considerable energy has gone into researching how surviving children compare with their peers. Academic success, self-esteem, behavioural difficulties, clumsiness, inattention, hyperactivity, anxiety . . . and ultimately their happiness . . . are all being formally studied. Of course, it is very difficult to un-muddle all the possible influences that might underlie a discrepancy between a heart child and his or her classmates. The origin might go right back to the mystery of what caused the heart problem in the first place (we know that for some children, the heart abnormality is only part of a wider issue in the genetic programming of a baby's development that may involve other organs including the brain.)* Or the basis might be inside the heart itself (even before birth, blood flow to the developing brain may be unusual in some way) or the operation (and the side effects of anaesthesia and heart-lung by-pass), the post-operative phase (when children may have a low blood pressure in the intensive care unit) or the family background (which influences academic achievement and behaviour in non-heart children). It turns out that most 'heart children' are functioning within a notional 'normal range' for most of the measurements so far made. However, it is also true that the *average* scores for their academic attainment, self-esteem, behavioural difficulties and so on are often a little worse than for children without heart problems – much as the *average* height of girls is lower than that of boys. Just as there are plenty of examples of particular girls being taller than particular boys, this does not preclude a particular heart child being top of their class. How does this help the parents of a survivor of cardiac surgery who is struggling academically or whose behaviour is difficult – what are they to believe? Their child's problems may or may not relate to their heart history. However, even though the labels 'dyslexia' or 'Attention Deficit Hyperactivity Disorder', 'autistic spectrum disorders' or 'learning difficulties' may not appeal, they are often a route to getting practical support – and it may help to motivate educational psychologists to assess a child with difficulties if they know that the child has had cardiac surgery.

* The commonest example is Down's syndrome; about one third of these children have cardiac abnormalities as well as their developmental delay. There are other 'syndromes' that affect many organs besides the heart (e.g. di George, CHARGE syndrome). We probably have a lot to learn about more subtle genetic influences.

The researchers are on the lookout for any clues that might offer opportunities for damage limitation. It is already pretty clear that having big operations behind them before children reach school age – and subsequently keeping them out of hospital – is a good investment for their future. Friendships unravel when a child is away from the classroom too much and, in surveys of contemporary children, having lost a lot of schooling is one of the strongest predictors of low scores when heart children assess their own 'quality of life'. (Oh the hurt of not being invited to children's parties.) Along with education and play, learning to make relationships is 'the work of childhood' and being away from school can impact all three.

After one of their number has survived a major operation, grateful families often raise money for medical research, including studies like these. But Christina has another suggestion for people to consider if they want to help heart children. In the mid 1990s, at the age of seven, she was offered a 'trip of a lifetime' by a charity. Christina had already had a Blalock shunt operation and subsequent serious surgery to close a hole in her heart and put in a tube to join her right ventricle to her pulmonary artery.* She had just emerged from a long and miserable hospital admission for an infection inside her heart when an envelope arrived in the post. Her doctors had nominated her for a 'Dreamflight'. She joined 250 children with all sorts of difficulties – some in wheelchairs, others with different medical contraptions – and over 100 volunteer carers, some Disney characters and a couple of television celebrities at a pre-flight party near London airport. Next day, they were driven to the decorated hangar of a private jumbo jet and were ferried up a fairy-tale archway into the plane and – hardly stopping to say goodbye to their parents – they all took off for Florida.

* Pulmonary atresia with Ventricular Septal Defect; the VSD was closed and a conduit/tube put in to jump the gap between right ventricle and pulmonary artery.

They had VIP treatment from start to finish. The Orange County police closed roads for their coaches; they visited all the theme parks and never once queued for a ride. 'I don't think any child felt out of place on the trip, everyone got on. It didn't matter what was wrong with you, what you looked like, nothing. It was ten days of feeling like a normal child without anyone making a fuss about anyone's illnesses; it was a week of pure bliss and fun!' Some children were terribly poorly, but the group had excellent medical cover and no limits were ever put on any child if they wanted to try something. The day they got home there wasn't a dry eye in the house; the trip had been transformative for Christina's confidence. As the charity's website says, 'Fun and joy are just as important as medical research and equipment.' Christina agrees, and hopes one day to volunteer to look after children on their own big trip.

★   ★   ★

Everyone who looks after children in hospital is awed by the way they just deal with whatever turns up. Most do not show the capacity for worry that engulfs their parents. Solidarity between families who meet on children's wards began with the outset of parental visiting and I have been told of letters going backwards and forwards between parents long after the death of one of the children. Formal 'support groups' emerged, usually clustered around particular hospitals, energized by these relationships. A mother told me: 'In 1970s Oklahoma, we did many things to support our doctors, nurses, and other families facing the same situations we had been in. We gained strength from each other. We held vigils with many families during surgeries, and shared our experiences with new "heart parents".' The internet has vastly extended the reach of these organizations. There is nobody better equipped to advise on the parenting of kids whose daily life may be undermined by their heart condition than experienced parents themselves; though they may try, doctors have little to offer in comparison. New in the past ten years or so, support groups organize

all-generation open days, catering for families drawn together by
their similar medical back-stories, or run virtual information services,
helplines, bulletin boards and Facebook groups. These have emerged
as wonderful resources for contemporary families. Though it is not
everyone's instinct to ask for – or give – advice, these support systems
have opened up a welcome sense of comradeship between people
who would not otherwise have contact with any one else with their
shared problem.

So what can neighbours, passers-by or teachers who wish these
heart children well do to help? When we were discussing this, one
man said ruefully – 'people know where they are with a wheelchair'. He is right. Cardiac 'disability' is largely invisible; we often
only notice when a child (or adult) fails to pick up speed when the
rest of us are in a hurry – a limitation so easily put down to laziness,
lack of 'fitness' or half-heartedness. Not realizing the cause, we rush
so quickly to judgement. Yet when the cause of a child's frustration
is understood, it is impossible not to feel respect for them and for
their efforts to appear 'normal'. Most of them have been through
more in their short lives that many of us have as adults, and they
have survived fears and setbacks. Their parents too deserve a trib-
ute. Here is one mother's point of view:

> I will always appreciate the desire and the actions to help
> and support that we received from friends and family (even
> when that advice and help wasn't all that helpful), because
> it was encouraging to know others cared, and worried. I
> will always appreciate the honesty (even when it was a bitter
> pill), compassion, and hope we received from our doctors
> and medical staff. I have even come to appreciate the lack
> of compassion we experienced on occasion, in that it taught
> me that in the end it was my fight, not others', to wage
> against the fear of 'what might happen'. If I have a regret,
> it is letting fear win the day far too many times in my life.

7
Going into hospital

In 1952, a forty-five-minute black-and-white film called *A Two-Year-Old Goes to Hospital* toured the Child Health meetings of Britain and later the whole English-speaking world. The camera observed a two-year-old child called Laura throughout her eight-day admission for an operation for an umbilical hernia. We see a confident little blonde girl arriving hand-in-hand with her mother being 'claimed' by apparently kindly nurses. We watch her mother's departure and the little girl's tears and distress as she is bathed, medicated and fed by strangers. Later we observe her dignified withdrawal from even kindly approaches, including those from her own mother when she visits. The recurrent explicit 'I want my mummy' gradually fades over the days, but her apparent composure is brittle. Towards the end of her stay a new toddler is admitted and cries. Laura is edgy but keeps her self-control saying, 'You're crying because you want your mummy. Don't cry.' Laura sits forlorn in her iron cot, clutching her teddy and her blanket. Frankly, the film makes difficult viewing.

This little film illustrates the atmosphere into which children were being admitted at the beginning of the story of cardiac surgery. Between then and now, the vibe of wards has changed, along with the mindsets of the staff, but let's not pretend that children do not still feel vulnerable, uncertain, scared – we can still see Laura's successors desolate and preternaturally withdrawn.

Parts of this chapter will amaze people familiar with modern hospitals. Children on adult wards? Parents visiting once a week? Screaming toddlers tied to their cots? Now, most children having heart surgery stay on wards that are reserved for cardiac cases. Family members come and go as they please. Often there are laundries, restaurant areas and hotel-style living spaces for parents. There are playrooms and schools. There are intensive care units and high-dependency units. Some hospitals have particular provision for teenagers, before they 'graduate' to adult services. The doctors, surgeons and nurses are all super-specialists with qualifications to prove it. But that is not how things were initially.

At the beginning, heart children shared clinics with children with a variety of other problems. If they came into hospital for an operation, many were cared for on grown-ups' wards. While their surgeons were only doing a few childhood heart operations each year, they spent most of their time dealing with adults' gall bladders, ulcers, hernias or lung cancers. It was not until hospitals realized that managing children's hearts could bring prestige and – in a fee-for-service environment – serious money, that the sort of specialist units emerged that we know today.

The USA was almost a decade ahead of Europe in making treatment available to its nation's children. After 1951, funding for surgery could come through a federal agency called the Children's Bureau. By 1952 there were five US states with regional centres for the diagnosis and treatment of congenital heart disease and the bureau liaised with them on behalf of out-of-state children. In practice, unless a family was very wealthy, this was the only way to get treatment. 'Doorstep cases' who simply showed up at the hospitals desperate or destitute had to appeal directly to the

President, or their Congressman – the Children's Bureau budget was always overspent.

As the specialty of paediatric cardiology emerged from the general looking-after of sick children, patients had to travel further and further to reach someone with up-to-date expertise. As a child in the 1940s and 1950s, one woman recalled her 200-mile travels with her mother to the Oklahoma 'Crippled Children's Hospital'. They would wait on benches in a big room hoping to be called in to see 'her' doctor – and might have to return the next day if her name had not come up. Another man, a four-year-old in 1954, remembered flying from Zanzibar and changing (propeller) planes at each leg of the journey, in Nairobi–Entebbe–Khartoum–Cairo–Rome–Paris–London to reach Guy's Hospital where he had a shunt operation (Brock had been at medical school with his grandfather). Still now, expertise is scattered and the price of specialism is that many patients have to travel enormous distances to get the care they need.

In the UK, many early child in-patients were accommodated on adult wards. In 1947, just who paid for Roy's hospitalization at the age of seven is unclear. Cardiac surgery had not come to England and there was still no National Health Service.* Post-war food rationing was still strict; his mother had to hand his ration book over to the hospital almoner. He had endocarditis, an infection somewhere inside his heart, and needed antibiotics. Penicillin was in very short supply and only available to the war-wounded

---

* The pamphlet distributed to every household in 1948 read: 'Your new National Health Service begins on 5 July. What is it? How do you get it? It will provide you with all medical, dental and nursing care. Everyone – rich or poor, man, woman or child – can use it or any part of it. There are no charges, except for a few special items. There are no insurance qualifications. But it is not a "charity". You are all paying for it, mainly as taxpayers, and it will relieve your money worries in time of illness.'

or through the auspices of a small committee of doctors. Roy's doctor must have pleaded his case and he arrived in a men's ward in Birmingham's spanking-new adult hospital, built largely with chocolate money.* He lingered there for six months as older men came and went.

Penicillin injections were given deep into muscle, which in a skinny boy meant into his bum. The needles had to be reused, and repeated resterilizing often made them blunt. Each injection was done in a kindly way, but the inescapable regime of injections four times each day for week after week must have felt brutal – Roy would watch the clock. His bottom became a mess of pock-marks, each spot chosen by Roy himself in a macabre game intended to shield both him and the commiserating nurses from the suffering of it all. In bed, he read to himself – the complete works of the 'Famous Five' – and sometimes the men nearby would come up with a bedtime story. If a nurse spotted that he looked dejected, she would carry him about on her hip. At night, whenever he turned over in bed, there was a reassuring light in the middle of the room. But for the kindness of nurses, it could all have been a lot worse. The entire medical and nursing staff made a great deal of fuss when he finally left the ward. Forty years later, when Roy had become a priest, he went back as their hospital chaplain. When I met him nearly seventy years after that long admission, Roy pulled a photo of the ward sister out of his wallet to show me. By way of telling me how tough the ordeal had been, he told me this story. Sitting quietly with a church prayer group that was meditating about martyrdom, he was listening to a parishioner reminiscing about the sufferings of a little boy on Ward East 2, whom she had

* Pre-NHS, the state was not paying for hospital-building. Chocolate was a big local industry and the chocolate families were philanthropic. Cadbury's bought the land and built the surgical wing; Terry's money paid for the medical wing.

looked after when she had been a nurse. 'Third bay on the left?' asked Father Roy.

Later, when cardiac surgery first became available to children in England, children were often admitted to the adult wards where their surgeons' other patients were accommodated. The expertise of the doctors and nurses there probably rendered the children safer than on a general children's ward – but it did mean that the child-patients were simply treated as little adults. (In 1964, when a wee Scottish girl told her mother excitedly, 'I'm going to the cinema tomorrow afternoon', the ward staff had probably thought they had done their job by telling the four-year-old that she was 'going to theatre' – the 'right word' is not enough, the job is not done unless the child understands.) In 1962 Barry was seven and quite enjoyed being a child on a men's ward. The hospital was next door to Wormwood Scrubs prison and the man in the next bed had murdered his wife – Barry remembers him as a nice bloke who chatted to him. In that era, the Hammersmith Hospital was one of the busiest cardiac surgical hospitals in England, yet Barry was there for almost six months after his Fallot repair and saw no more than a dozen other children. Where were his all contemporaries born with heart disease – the sorts of children who fill the wards now? In brief, most of them were dead. Only a small proportion of 'operable' children found their way to services that could help them, and for those with difficult problems – valves, ventricles or blood vessels missing – 1960s hospitals had nothing to offer and their hearts just failed.

As children's heart surgery became established through the 1950s, 1960s and 1970s, a move into dedicated children's facilities became the norm on both sides of the Atlantic. The paradoxical upshot of that shift was a regimented and often intransigent separation of the children from their parents. At a time when admitting a child to hospital in Africa or India without a family member would have been unheard of, in most English and American hospitals a young child might see its mother for a couple of hours each week – and medical regimes often mandated very long hospital admissions. Up until the late 1950s, most British and American hospitals required a wholesale handover of all children to the hospital nursing staff. Babies were handled only when necessary, food not taken at one feeding time was not made up at the next, whining children were ignored on principle. While he was on the men's ward, Roy's nurses had been allowed to console him if he was miserable and his mother could visit every day; this would never have happened on a children's ward at the time.

What was going on? Justifications for minimizing parental involvement on hospital wards were couched in the language of science, but arguably the subtext was about power-sharing. The hospital ward had always been the nurses' domain; the visit of a senior doctor might have been the big event of the day, but even he was the 'guest' of the senior nurse. In both the UK and USA in the 1950s, nurses were necessarily single, childless women who were required to live in accommodation attached to the hospitals. They deferred to authority in their personal as well as their working lives, much like their male contemporaries who were conscripted to military service were required to do. There was no ambiguity about their relationship to children – it was strictly professional – and routine was very much the order of the day. Inviting parents into a children's ward was largely the prerogative of the nursing hierarchy, and they really did not want to negotiate.

There were also practicalities. To understand why a nurse might tie a distressed child's leg to the bars of the cot rather than simply pick her up, we need also to appreciate what a nurse had to do in a day's work. At a time when the Minneapolis doctors were wowing the world with the news of the first successful Fallot repair, Minneapolis nurses were sewing newspapers together with old sheets over them to put under children liable to soil the bed-clothes. A junior nurse's role in London in the same era was also mainly menial; she was not allowed to sit down – not even during the handover reports between shifts. Wards had coal fires (nurses' job), nurses had to cook the breakfasts (eggs and kippers would arrive unprepared from the kitchens),* beds had to be made,† vomit bowls washed, cloth nappies soaked, lockers cleaned. Bed-rest was very commonly prescribed, which meant bedpans and bed baths. 'Patient observations' (pulse, temperature, breathing rate) needed charting for every patient every few hours using glass thermometers and a watch. In the ward side-room, nurses had to sterilize injection syringes and needles and cut their own gauze squares to use as swabs. To be fair, this regime did not permit the 'luxury' of cuddling a distressed toddler. If parents were to visit, the additional workload of tidying-up before and cleaning up after had to be considered – and what about the germs coming in from the streets?

The fact that nurses already had a gruelling routine did not, of course, make it any less distressing for the children, and this is why the film about Laura became so important. Behind the camera was James Robertson, a psychiatric social worker from the Tavistock Clinic in London. During the Second World War, he had been a conscientious objector, remaining in London ostensibly to maintain the boilers of the Hampstead Wartime Nurseries, which were presided over by a lady called Anna Freud.‡ The nursery itself was funded by the American Foster Parents Plan for War Children and took in almost 100 children – mainly under-threes – who had been separated from their families during the London Blitz. Throughout the social chaos, the V2 rockets landing nearby, the trips down to the Underground air-raid shelters and the occasional visits of

---

* Brains for those on a 'light diet'.
† Every day: rubber sheet underneath, top sheet moved to become the bottom sheet, new top-sheet, new pillow case; the precision of the bed-sheet corners was independently inspected.
‡ Daughter of Sigmund.

family members, Robertson observed the profound unhappiness of these children – most of whom were too young to have much verbal language – as they coped with the absence of their parents.

In peacetime, he continued to study the behaviour of children separated from their parents and discerned a similar battlefield on the children's wards of hospitals. The documentary was produced as an attempt at scientific objectivity, giving anyone a chance to make up their own minds. For the film, Laura had been chosen at random by a hospital clerk and the times when the camera would be turned on were agreed in advance.* The film compelled medical staff to reconsider the significance of a child's non-verbal communication. It was distributed as a shock tactic, and the discussions it provoked served that purpose.

Many doctors and nurses received it with blatant hostility. Medical staff contested Robertson's inference in the film that the hospitalized children were profoundly unhappy. They pointed out how quiet and 'well behaved' they would eventually become in their parents' absence and how distressed children were when their mothers visited. How was a cardiac nurse to keep a child's heart rate low with all this agitation going on? The debates about ward childcare policies raged between factions of hospital staff; parents' views were immaterial and children's completely irrelevant. Discussing the dispute about increasing visiting hours in an American nursing article in the 1950s, the author laid out the facts of the matter: increasing parental visiting hours increased the work for the nurses. Nobody disputed this; it was simply true that visiting hours really did have a troublesome aftermath and even if nurses recognized the cause of the child's distress, that did not make it any easier to get

---

* Robertson's research grant only funded the purchase of eighty minutes' worth of cine film and the final cut is forty-five minutes long. He had never used a camera before, so it is easy to believe that Robertson must have included almost all of the usable footage.

medicines or food into tearful children – and this was to happen every day rather than just once each week?

Over the next twenty years, ward regimes changed gradually, starting with extending visiting hours.* Later, some forward-thinking head nurses began to experiment with the notion that 'standards' could be allowed to slip a little more. Might some mothers somehow be accommodated within the ward, perhaps in the few two-bed and single rooms available – they might even lighten the load? (A 1951 medical article noted that a mother sharing care of her child 'needs little or no off-duty time, as the sleep requirements of a mother fall to near zero when her own child is acutely ill'.) However, this scheme was not an overnight success for either nurses or parents – and arguably tensions continue even now.

A 1969 UK-based article, 'The Captive Mother', documented an overtly adversarial atmosphere on children's wards where mutual criticism could blow up over a dirty nappy; a mother felt patronized by a childless nurse criticizing her nappy-folding technique while a nurse felt censured over a medicine given five minutes late. Then as now, a nurse's professional skill with needles, medicines and technology can seem to trump a mother's capacity to look after her own child – just at a time when they are the absolute focus of all her love and attention. Another medical article called 'No Thanks, I'd Rather Stay at Home' documented the reasons that 400 mothers gave for declining an offer of a bed near their hospitalized child. As nowadays, the most common reason was having to balance the needs of other children at home – as well as 'I've got to do my husband's meals' and 'I don't like hospitals' and 'I'd be no good at it'. But gradually on both sides of the Atlantic, hospital wards felt their way forwards and a perkier film, *Going to Hospital with Mother*,

---

* In 1952, 23 per cent of children's wards allowed daily visiting; in 1964 it was 83 per cent.

was made in 1958 in the first English hospital ward to regularly accommodate mothers at their children's bedsides.

By the time I joined the specialty, ward regimes had softened appreciably, but I knew there had been a battle. In her 1965 novel *The Millstone*,* set partly in the (thinly disguised) Great Ormond Street Hospital in London, Margaret Drabble describes the ferocity of a mother's fight for access to her cardiac child. (The battle-lines had been drawn between a mother and a ward sister; the sympathetic medical consultant was anxious not to take sides.)

Anyone who can remember being in hospital alone at a young age might be advised to think twice before watching the little film about Laura; it is certain to evoke complex emotions. But each of the people who dredged up fragments of hospital memories for me decades later had managed somehow, and could look back and reflect. Carol was only three in 1972 but clearly remembers standing at the door of the ward during the so-called 'rest period' screaming, 'I don't want you, I want my mummy.' As her mother said goodbye, she would make her leave her wedding ring and purse behind as a pledge that she would ever return. One visiting-time, while she was sitting on her father's knee as he read to her, a nurse arrived with some medicines. Carol refused to cooperate. The nurse picked her up bodily, took her to the bathroom, forced the medicines down and sent her father home: these memories still burn decades later – as does the triumph of biting that same nurse the following day. Carol went home after her operation, drew scars on her dolls and grew up to be a children's nurse. On one ward round, wondering what to do about a child crying after a heart operation, a young doctor pronounced, 'Anyway, children don't feel pain.' He won't forget Carol's put-down: 'Have you? . . . I have.'

---

* 'But who so shall offend one of these little ones who believe in me, it were better that a millstone were hanged about his neck and that he were drowned in the depth of the sea' (Matthew 18:6).

Susan spent months in hospital in the late 1950s and remembers having mixed feelings about her mother's weekly visits; there were definitely no tears when it came to saying goodbye. In retrospect, she felt resigned to the abandonment. Her ward had beds down each side with tall windows so she could watch the sky. There was a working model-railway in the middle of the ward and a table in the corner where she might be allowed out of bed to have tea. There was always a nurse in the room. The routine did not vary. She was woken very early with a drink and her bed made before she was tucked in tightly again for Matron's inspection. Breakfast involved boiled eggs. Through all the bed-baths she never felt 'invaded' by the nurses; not so the doctors, who imposed a very 'veterinary' relationship with their child-patients. Susan remembers being stood up, aged eight, completely naked while a large group of doctors talked about her and measured her. She wet herself in distress but nobody noticed. A very cross nurse came and mopped her up. At the time, Susan thought the nurse was vexed with her, but in retrospect it was probably with the crass doctors. The months of seeing her mother only for a Sunday afternoon currant-bun left her with a feeling of abandonment that pervaded her childhood and adolescence. Decades later she and her husband fostered children from broken families.

Rita was six when in 1955 when she was admitted to a Boston hospital for a catheterization. During that admission, Rita shared a side-room with a little girl who was only three and completely inconsolable. The toddler cried incessantly, but no mother and no nurse ever appeared. Like Laura in the film, Rita empathized with the younger child and spent the whole day doing her six-year-old best to cuddle and console her and exhausted herself trying. Once the baby was asleep, Rita woke up to her own uncertain situation and started weeping herself. Now looking back as a grandmother, 'barbaric' is the word Rita uses to describe the exclusion of her little companion's parents.

Our dismay about these children's experiences presupposes that they had left a secure family environment, but four-year-old Patrick thrived on his 1960s ward. Getting away from the squalor of his tenement home was like 'turning on a light bulb'.* He thought he had seen his first television (it turned out to be an aquarium), he ate his first tomato, he smelled new smells. More important, the ward offered a whole different way of being – the day had a routine, a regular supply of delicious food, conversations; at home children had to put up and shut up.

For many children, the 'work of the day' would involve needles – injections or blood tests. Many remember a room halfway along the ward where they would 'do things to kids'. Others tell of how the sight of the phlebotomist entering the ward with her trolley to take blood made all the children start to cry at once. Ward rounds are remembered, sometimes with hilarity. Ranking the doctors (the longer the white coat, the more senior the doctor) was easier than decoding the meaning of nurses' veils and sleeve lengths and aprons and uniform colours. Rounds involved much shifting of screens and wheeling of trollies and shuffling of notes and shouting at medical students. Nothing much was said to a child – 'They talked about me like I was a side of beef,' said one man.

★   ★   ★

The notion of 'protecting' children by silence is a fiction mainly perpetuated by adults to protect themselves from their own discomfort and distress (in my humble opinion). One patient stated the problem quite clearly for me when she said, 'Events that would be considered traumatic for a child in any other walk of life are assumed benign when they occur within a medical setting in the name of saving a life.' She is right: in any other context, strangers

---

* The nurses kept him in for medically unnecessary months because they couldn't bear to send him home to his shambles.

restraining a child and doing painful things to them would be completely out of order, even legally abusive, and nothing prepares a child brought up in a close and loving family for that experience. They deserve every possible support in dealing with the experience – and that is hard for everyone.

One of the reasons it seems so hard for very young children to be in hospital without a parent is because they rely so much on physical comforting and the reassurance of a protective parental presence; explanations do not cut much ice with a two-year-old. But by the time children are talkative most are curious and take pleasure in asking the reasons for things. At nursery, they stray away from their parents and begin to rely on their own resources. If they are not given any understanding of why unfamiliar people are doing alarming and horrible things to them, young children often think they are being punished for some baffling misdemeanour.

Sian entered hospital a very knowledgeable little four-year-old. Her mother was a primary school teacher and to prepare her daughter she used the Ladybird picture book called *The Nurse*. For Sian, this had the virtue of a cover picturing a little girl wearing a rather fetching red coat being helped indoors by a solicitous nurse with a fascinating veil. The book explained the job of a nurse, the role of a child in the routine of a ward, helpful facts about tests, about going to sleep for operations, about visiting and about going home. For Sian, everything turned out 'as advertised' – the relationship with the nurses was starched and formal, just as in the book. Fortuitously, one picture had even shown a black nurse – and on the ward was a real black nurse (an eye-opening experience for a child brought up in a 1960s English coastal town). Sian's mother was not able to visit every day (work, long journey, another child) but her daughter managed happily, largely thanks to preparation.

Bernhard's experience was a complete contrast; in his home there had always been an embargo on difficult conversations. Even in 1961, when he was thirteen and heading for his second operation, the purpose of the long journey to London was not discussed at all. His mother had been a Jehovah's Witness – she used to push him around as she was proselytizing; the 'right thing to do' was not a subject of opinion or discussion. Perhaps only his father had acquiesced to surgery. It took years before Bernhard stopped holding the deception against his mother.

Gradually doctors and nurses came to recognize the virtue of preparing children for their forthcoming experiences. Play is a natural way to check out what children understand about what is happening to them and 'play staff', who never did anything nasty to patients, were often co-opted to explain forthcoming operations to children, using puppets or pictures or elaborate dolls' hospitals. Children and parents might be invited to visit a ward or an intensive care unit as part of an out-patient visit so they can see other children and families coping before they have to themselves. If everyone's primary focus is to minimize their child's distress, they need to keep their own terror under control; they are in charge of the hugs and often have to be very creative to keep the lines of communication open.

To be fair, a particular child's 'need to know' is very difficult to gauge on the fly and no child can be perfectly prepared for every eventuality. This makes it even more important that patients can feel able to ask questions and be answered with – some sort of – truth; even children have bullshit-detectors. When Richard was admitted to an adult ward for his operation when he was thirteen, he really liked the way his surgeon talked him through his aortic valve operation in a grown-up way. Richard knew that some people died, but looking around the much older people on the ward, he figured that it wasn't going to be him. The downside of being with the grown-ups was that the food rations seemed very meagre. On the night before his operation, the lady opposite took pity and offered him her own supper. Richard had noticed her apprehension and later enquired after her and was told she had 'gone to another ward'. After his operation, Richard returned to a single room with a bathroom shared with one other cubicle. Needing a wee, he pushed open the bathroom door and found his neighbour cold and stiff on the floor – another one who had 'gone to another ward'.*

★　★　★

In the lifetime of congenital heart surgical treatment, changes in ward layouts and the very presence of parents has transformed the ambience of wards. But nothing has evolved more than the relationship between nurses and doctors. A Minnesota nurse of the 1950s tells how a bevvy of nurses would vacate a lift if doctors wanted to get in – it's unimaginable that that would happen now! A Great Ormond Street Hospital consultant of the 1950s said that his hospital turned out second-class nurses but first-class cleaners;† that was my own hospital. By the time I arrived there twenty years later, nurses were no longer 'handmaidens' to the doctors and one taught me all the practical paediatrics I know. From being 'cleaners' in the 1950s, they now manage complex equipment and have levels of responsibilities for patients' safety comparable to air-traffic controllers' (without the hike in pay). In certain units, both nurses and doctors wear scrubs; some doctors are female and some nurses male – so unless the professionals introduce themselves, it can be very difficult for newcomers to know to what category of person they are talking.

---

* Another euphemism patients remember is 'gone to Rose Cottage'.
† One man who had been a boy on an adult ward in another hospital remembers that maintaining spanking cleanliness was the nurses' job during the week, but on Sundays the whole place would be scoured by a line-up of delightful black orderlies who arrived, turned on the radiogram and played Motown as they worked, teasing and delighting everyone; hearing Aretha Franklin takes him straight back to those days.

For the children, there are still needles, but not nearly so many. More than half of all childhood operations are undertaken before the children are even one year old; the experience is unforgettable for their parents, but for the children the admission is just another family story. The concept of 'convalescence' has long gone, along with long hospital stays 'for observation' – as soon as they are well enough, children are sent home.

Other aspects of hospitals have not changed so much. It remains true that nurses are the locals who enforce the laws and speak the language of hospital wards. When they first arrive, mothers have no more authority or knowledge than visitors from another country. Depending on the atmosphere of the ward, they might be welcomed or snubbed like unwanted immigrants. Is a parent 'allowed' to sleep near their child, to be present while a medical round is conferring, to watch a team try to resuscitate their child? The balance of power between nurses and parents changes at different rates for different reasons in different wards in different hospitals in different countries.

Academics have interviewed 1950s and 1960s nurses about their apparent emotional detachment from the children for whom they were caring. In tape-recorded oral histories, some ex-nurses became very upset as they recalled the worst excesses of what they had colluded with; one even referred to episodes that were 'like a concentration camp'.* Others regarded their emotional neutrality as perfectly 'correct', saying that it was important to treat all children the same and crucial not to get 'emotionally involved' with their patients if they were to do their core job properly. Many doctors and nurses are still ready with the assertion that emotional neutrality defends them from being overwhelmed, though their

---

* A nurse's description of being obliged to hold children down while her colleague cut off their eyelashes before eye operations was the one that stayed with me!

argument implicitly acknowledges the extent of the suffering that they observe every day.

Those same 'don't get too involved' professionals are not always ready with suggestions as to whose job it is to support a distressed child in their care. It is true that the path between avoiding one's own burnout while remaining open to a child's anguish is a delicate one to tread, but many nurses and doctors really do care – and some have the gift of being both 'professional' and warm. Such nurses are often remembered with great affection as their child-patients grow up: Sister Mann, Megan, 'Sooty', Adelaide, Sister Sherwood, Ellen and Eleanor, Sister Asquith, Florence Mary – all 'mentioned in dispatches' by patients decades later.

★   ★   ★

Typically, the evening before an operation the time comes for parents to meet the surgeon who will put a knife to their child's chest the next day. Part of the surgeon's agenda is to get some paperwork signed.

If someone in the street plunges a knife into your child, a criminal offence has occurred; the person with the weapon becomes the perpetrator and the victim has recourse to the law – in most jurisdictions this involves the Laws of Battery. The very earliest surgeons realized that they were in a legally vulnerable position, and from the Middle Ages historical archives hold documents composed by surgeons and signed by their patients before an operation. Given the desperate diseases and desperate measures involved, operations commonly ended badly, making the surgeons' insistence on being exonerated in advance seem completely understandable. This early 'red tape' anticipated the documents that are used today to underwrite the lawful justification for operations; they are the surgeon's legal defence against a claim of 'Battery'.

During the 1900s, as surgery began to make a real impact on the lives of sick people, these wholesale waivers of responsibility did not satisfy the courts when legal disputes arose over who was liable for post-operative complications. Gradually the law clarified several notions. First, it was stipulated that patients had the right to expect their surgeons to be adequately trained to undertake the planned operation (this remains a real problem for some rare congenital heart operations where there are too few cases for practice to make perfect). Second, the law clarified that the decision about what is in the 'best interests' of a patient lies unequivocally with an (adult) patient himself – even if the surgeon feels he 'knows better'; when the patient is a child, both the parents and the specialist team have legal duties to work for the child's 'best interests' and they occasionally disagree. Finally the courts have asserted that a patient's agreement to an operation only holds in law if they have an understanding of its risks as well as its benefits, including some grasp of alternative choices. It is honouring the last of these provisos – the need for 'informed consent' – that has been the most bothering requirement in practice. It can seem difficult for doctors to second-guess just how much information a particular patient really wants or understands. A few patients might choose to study all the 'small print', while others, if only they were able to close their ears to the bad stuff, would prefer to opt out of the burden of responsibility.*

What often happens in practice is that just before an operation, when bullet-proof optimism might be so much more comfortable for the people on both sides of the parent–surgeon conversation, an explicit plan has to be agreed, and serious words like 'death' and 'brain damage' have somehow to be blurted out. In practice, it should be unusual for parents to get as far as this conversation

---

* My own thought is that if the 'surgical contract' were being written from scratch in the modern era, it might have been better to put the initiative with the patient and require them to *request* the surgeon to operate, rather than the surgeon to ask the patient to *consent* to their plan.

without a reasonable understanding of what lies ahead, and most approach these discussions completely ready to sign. For the mothers and fathers of some newborns, the alternative to surgery is their baby's certain and imminent death, while surgery offers a hope that is not completely hopeless; in those situations most of us would sign almost anything.

But from the parents' point of view, signing the paper is not the main purpose of the meeting; they mainly want to size up the guy to whom they are about to trust their child's life. Though surgeons commonly explain the steps of the operation, often drawing diagrams on scraps of paper, most parents appreciate this more as evidence that *the surgeon* knows how to do the operation – an exhibition of self-confidence – rather than a detailed lesson that *they* need to grasp. Senior surgeons will probably have sat through a few thousand consent conversations and may be tempted to delegate the job to very junior staff. But without actually meeting him (or her), the parents do not get their part of the bargain so, apart from exceptional circumstances, it is the main surgeon who conducts the formalities. The papers are signed and, as if a referee's whistle had blown for play to stop, everyone jumps up and leaves. Everybody is committed.

8
Magic sleep

You feel a cold sensation as fluid goes in. Then you are
told to 'count down from 10' and only manage a couple
of numbers, but some consciousness lingers for a few
moments after that. There is a sense of being committed,
of no going back. A feeling of pressure in your ears like
when you are swimming underwater, and a rushing roar,
a bit like when aeroplane engines gear up before take-off,
sort of overwhelming. Then you reach some sort of tipping
point after which you sink into yourself. It's powerful,
almost sublime, not frightening. Then with absolutely no
sense of the passing of time, the light opens up again like
in Looney Tunes cartoon, and you are in another place.

(Thanks to Guy for this description.)

Nobody underrates the audacity of open-heart surgery
in children but a surgeon is at least able to explain the
whole procedure. He can reduce it to steps involving pipes, pumps,
valves, stitches and patches, so that you can come to understand it
in the same terms as tackling a rather complicated central heating
repair. Talk in the same way to an anaesthetist, and what she does
sounds like a conjuring trick. You are put into a coma, you can't

feel, you can't move, you can't breathe, you are not afraid. And when it's all over, the coma is reversed, responsibility for your breathing and movement is handed back to you and you wake up remembering nothing. That is modern magic.

In charge of this uncanny closing-down of your consciousness, the last person you see, the one a parent entrusts their child to, is the anaesthetist. One wag said that anaesthetists are in charge of the trickiest parts of an operation – the take-off and landing – while the surgeon just deals with the in-flight entertainment. Anaesthesia is the ultimate multi-tasking job. While the surgeon is dealing with what is going on in the big hole in the chest, someone else needs to keep the patient asleep, watch all the screens and keep track of a spreadsheet of all the blood, fluids and drugs going in and out of the body. They need technical skills to get tubes into the tiny veins, arteries and airways of very small babies. When everything is going smoothly, anaesthetists are taken for granted. When things are about to go wrong – like the bomb squad, they are the ones to defuse the situation. When everything is going to hell in a handbag, they need to be an oasis of calm and decisiveness. And they also need to be sweet to their patients.

Almost all parents are chronically anxious; in everyday life, many barely let a young child out of their sight. Whether in the 1940s or in the 2014s, a parent handing a child over for a cardiac operation feels a big tug – one mother called its physicality a 'G-force'. Just where and when these final kisses happen has changed over the years as most hospitals gradually relaxed their unwritten rules about parents' presence – but their involvement started from zero.

In 1955, Rita sat in the back of the car on the trip from Rhode Island to Boston, playing; her parents were very tense. She was seven and thought it was just another hospital visit. Her mother and father were not permitted to see her on the day of her surgery. Looking back from her middle age, Rita told me she remembered lying on some sort of trolley and being pushed across a glass walk-way from one part of the hospital to another – from the ward to the operating room. Unbeknown to her at the time, her parents were sitting in the parking lot below, watching the passage of the gurney. They had been told Rita's chances of survival were 50:50.

The embargo on parents being near their children was begin-ning to loosen by the time Carol was operated in England in the 1970s. Her mother was allowed to accompany her as she sat bolt upright, wide awake on the trolley heading for the operating room. As they approached the heavy plastic swing doors, her mother was turned away. To say that Carol screamed is an understatement. A nurse scooped her up and carried her straight into the operating room, saying, 'Stop being a naughty girl.' She was only three and a half.

Gradually parents were allowed nearer and nearer the action and the art of 'premedication' also improved – now children having planned operations are given some sort of sedative so that they are sleepy for their journey. Even if their child falls fast asleep in their ward bed, many parents want to bear witness to their child's story for as long as they can. It's quite a stunt to watch as an anaesthetist sets to work with needles and mask and a child fails to count to ten. Viewing the performance may make it easier for a parent to walk away, confident in someone with syringes and 'superpowers' – though 'you are in the best possible hands' may have lost its power to reassure, since it has become a cliché for something about to go terribly wrong in TV hospital soaps. Not all anaesthetists are immune to the extra pressure of being observed while doing their job, and it is not necessarily easy for parents either – one father was spooked for years by the memory of leaving his son behind while he was being 'smothered' with an oxygen mask. These days, many children are operated at an age when nobody would expect them to remember anything, but the innermost experience of parents has hardly changed over the years. No amount of reassurance can

eliminate the thought that they might not see their child alive
again. If it were an opera and not an operation, the soprano would
be singing a long, sad aria as she walked away from an anaesthetic room.

★   ★   ★

Some date the very first congenital heart operation to 1938, when
a seven-year-old girl called Lorraine in Boston had an operation
to tie off a 'ductus'. The ductus is a vessel inside the chest but outside the heart; part of the normal circulation in the womb, it can
become a problem if it fails to close after birth. Speaking years later
as a great-grandmother, Lorraine recalls that her mother was simply
required to drop her off at the hospital and then leave. On the day
of surgery, she remembered being laid directly on the operating
table surrounded by masked, white-gowned surgeons and nurses
and – looming above them – spectators' faces gazing at her from
the gallery, a child caught like a rabbit in headlights.

For the first congenital heart operations, children were put
to sleep and kept asleep with a gas, usually ether. This was given
through a rubber mask, much like one an aviator might wear in the
movies. Corrugated tubing connected the front of the mask to a
contraption that maintained reasonable proportions of oxygen and
sleepy gas in the breathing circuit; it incorporated a squishy black
latex bag that allowed the anaesthetist to puff up the pressure in
the lungs a little. There was no 'breathing machine' and the anaesthetist could not 'take over' for more than a few inefficient puffs
if a child stopped breathing for herself. 'Monitoring' was with a
finger on a pulse (speeding up or slowing down presaged trouble).
Thermometers were made of glass. Blood oxygen levels could
not be checked. Nothing was electric, nothing was digital, there
were no monitor screens. If anything went wrong, chest compressions for cardiac arrest had not been invented, nor pacemakers,
nor defibrillators.

For Lorraine's ductus-closure operation in 1938, her 'anaesthetist' was a nurse called Betty Lank. She had needed to shrink an
adult-sized gas mask in alcohol to make it fit sufficiently tightly over
the child's face and Lorraine had to breathe for herself throughout
the operation. Once asleep, she was laid on her right side and
her left arm draped over her head to expose the left side of her
chest. Using one hand to keep the gas mask firmly over Lorraine's
nose and mouth, her anaesthetic nurse used her other hand alter-
nately to keep a little pressure on the squeeze bag and to check
Lorraine's pulse with a finger on the artery in front of her ear.
Aiming between her ribs, the surgeon cut through into her chest,
nudged her left lung out of his way, found her ductus and tied a
tape around it. After the operation the mask came off, Lorraine
woke up and was wheeled off to the ward.

The surgeon had been a Dr Gross and he had waited for his
boss to go on holiday because he had been expressly forbidden to
carry out the operation. But the prospect of fame had beckoned;
this had been an operation that many had talked about but few
had dared to do. The previous year, a child at another hospital had
died five days after closure of an infected duct. Lorraine's surgeon
had been quick and the team had been lucky. Years later he told
Lorraine, 'If you hadn't survived, I'd now be a chicken farmer in
Vermont.' Now, closing a ductus is 'the appendicectomy of heart
operations'.

By her own account, the nurse anaesthetist had been 'scared to
death, scared to death' – and rightly. What horrifies a contemporary
anaesthetist hearing about these arrangements was the reliance on
that gas mask. It needed to be leak-proof to avoid the sleepy-gas
escaping, the anaesthetic lightening and the child waking up and
moving while the surgeon was doing something crucial deep in
her chest – and what if the nurse had got cramp in her hand? Also,
it was absolutely necessary that the patient breathed for herself
throughout the operation, including the time when one side of

her chest was open to the air – because the anaesthetist had no way of taking over if the breathing stopped. Our rib cages protect our lungs from the pressure of the atmosphere. When the left side of Lorraine's chest was open, her left lung must have collapsed, squashed by atmospheric pressure, leaving her breathing only with her right (lower) lung. What if that had been insufficient?

The very first Blalock operations in the mid 1940s also used ether as the anaesthetic agent, dripped on to some gauze over the child's nose and mouth; the lesson that this arrangement was inherently unsafe was learned through the deaths of many children. Marilyn's first operation in 1947 was at the Crippled Children's Hospital in Oklahoma. She showed me a cutting from the local newspaper which jubilantly recorded a 'double operation' explaining 'the baby's strength was not equal to the ordeal of one exceedingly lengthy operation'. Rubbish. In fact the surgeons had lost their nerve when she collapsed during the first anaesthetic; they sewed her up quickly and took her back to the ward, prob- ably thinking she would die. They tried again a week later and this time the shunt connection was achieved and Marilyn survived her 'near-miss' (but for years she associated going through the doors of that hospital with the smell of ether).

For safety's sake, one major thing had to change. To give them control of the patient's breathing, the anaesthetists would put a tube into the child's mouth, down his throat, past his vocal cords and into his windpipe; it takes experience and a deeply anaesthetized or paralysed child to achieve this. But once this 'endotracheal tube' is secured in the right place and attached to the anaesthetic circuit, the anaesthetist is in control and if necessary can himself puff gas and oxygen into the patient's lungs.

By the mid 1950s, the gas being delivered was cyclopropane. Cyclopropane had the merit of being sweet-smelling and quite potent – a few deep breaths would put a patient 'under' but had the major disadvantage of being explosive. Like in the school experiment, an explosion needs a fuel, some oxygen and some heat. The fuel (the flammable anaesthetic gas) and the oxygen were ready-mixed in the anaesthetic circuit and the extensive list of things that have provided the igniting heat have included: diathermy (a surgeon's gadget that cuts and seals small blood vessels), electrical plugs, a static spark from silk underwear, an anaesthetist's cigarette. Anaesthetic explosions often caused more annoyance than injury, but severe destruction and deaths of patients, surgeons and anaesthetists have all been recorded.* Anaesthetic explosions have all but died out with the change in gases used and attention to operating-room safety.

Even with a tube in the windpipe, anaesthetizing early patients for a Blalock-Taussig shunt must have been an extremely nerve-wracking experience. Pioneering teams felt obliged to offer surgery to any child who might possibly benefit, because the child's deterioration and death were otherwise inevitable. This meant that some of the children were – as a modern anaesthetist might say – 'hardly fit for a haircut'. These patients were already blue and in precarious health because of low blood flow to the lungs. The plan was to supplement the lung-blood flow in the long term by surgically diverting some blood from an arm artery and plugging it into the lung artery to increase its blood supply. The problem was that to even find the relevant arteries, the surgeon needed to open one side of the chest, squashing the lung on that side and making oxygen levels worse rather than better in the short term. Unfortunately some patients 'could not take the anaesthetic' and

* The last death from an anaesthetic explosion recorded in England was in 1954. There was a loud bang, bits of equipment flew about and smoke was seen coming from the patient's mouth. The operation took place at night when the atmosphere in the theatres was less humid than during the day because there was no steam from the sterilisers. The patient's widow sued the anaesthetist but (in a first for the UK) the Hospital Board was found to be negligent.

their hearts stopped before the crucial part of the operation had got underway.* Even the fact that the heart had stopped often took some time to recognize – it depended on the anaesthetist keeping a finger on an already faint and thready pulse or occasionally running a short strip of ECG tracing to check the heart's rhythm.

During the 1950s and 1960s, the operations became more ambitious as the era of 'open-heart surgery' began. Though the preferred drug cocktails have varied over the years, the essential brief of the anaesthetist has stayed the same: to keep the patient asleep and still, free of pain and stable. Different drugs are used to deliver unconsciousness, immobility, pain relief and (if necessary) to push the blood pressure up or down, so a cardiac anaesthetist goes to work with an impressive arsenal of syringes and ampoules. Running at least ten interacting drugs, anaesthetists have a lot to juggle.

After a child is handed over to an anaesthetist's care and before the surgeon first applies scalpel to skin, the first task is to put the child to sleep. Going-to-sleep drugs come as gases or liquids; the gases must be inhaled, the liquids need to be injected into veins. The liquids work astonishingly quickly but need a needle; for many children this is not the ideal way of slipping off quietly, so gases are still used.

'Sleep' is a euphemism for the state of unconsciousness of a cardiac surgical patient – what kind of 'sleep' would last through a saw opening your chest? The stages of anaesthesia are classed according to depth. As 'anaesthesia' is established, the patient progresses through stages 1-2-3, and on return to consciousness the steps reverse as 3-2-1. (There is a fourth stage, but nobody plans to go there.) Though you will not find the steps described like this in any textbook, a recovery room nurse explains them as '1: aphrodisia,

---

* In Blalock's first 500 shunts, more than one in twenty children had a cardiac arrest before the arteries had been prepared for joining up.

2: even dizzier, 3: deep and 4: dicey'. Stage 1 describes a happy state
of altered consciousness when patients may still talk; during induc-
tion – 'on the way down' – children may say daft and endearing
things; 'on the way up', middle-aged men might propose marriage
to recovery-room nurses.* Stage 2 is a brief period of excitement
before stage 3 supervenes, the muscles relax, breathing becomes
shallow and steady; the patient is 'deep' and ready for surgery.
Overshoot to stage 4 and the impulse to breathe is depressed, the
circulation becomes troublesome and heart action is precarious:
overdose, 'dicey'.

A patient will be 'relaxed' as they 'sleep', but 'relaxation' under
anaesthesia is just another euphemism. The operating field has to
be absolutely still if a surgeon is to have a realistic chance of being
able to sew one small blood vessel to another. But from the anaesthetist's point of view, stopping one movement means stopping
them all, including the muscles that power a patient's breathing.
Medical people call this process 'paralysing the patient' – deliberately rendering them completely unable to move – 'relaxing' does
sound less scary. Either way, the anaesthetist needs to take over
complete responsibility for puffing air into the lungs. In the early
years they would 'hand-ventilate', squeezing the black rubber bag
in the anaesthetic circuit and pushing gas and oxygen through the
tube in the trachea and into the lungs. As the operations got longer
and longer, anaesthetists were pleased to have machines to do the
squeezing, available from the mid 1950s.

Neither the drugs that cause the 'relaxation' nor those that
maintain the 'sleep' do much for the pain of the scalpels and saws.
Fortunately, there have been good pain-killing drugs available to
medicine for hundreds of years, and in the early days of heart
surgery the poppy-derived opiates did a good job of preventing
pain during an operation. But since the drugs for keeping still,

* http://www.johnpowell.net/gasman/

for blocking pain and for blotting out awareness are all different, it is conceivable that the 'keeping-still' and the 'pain-killing' drugs could be working while the 'staying asleep' drugs are not. This is rare but possible. It sounds scary, but here are the only accounts I have heard of how it feels.

In the early 1990s in London, a five-year-old was having a tricky operation attempting to streamline her rather exotic lung-blood supply. Over twenty years later, she remembers a queer feeling: she could not even open her eyes but was in no pain. Her sense that she was properly conscious was confirmed by a disembodied voice saying, 'Oh crap, she's awake' – then nothing! In 1973 in Birmingham, Alabama, another child's experience was more complex. She was twelve and having an open-heart operation that was not going smoothly. She sensed her body suspended above the operating table, looking down at the doctors doing surgery on her. Towards the end of the operation she heard one of the doctors say, 'We almost lost her.' As they were wheeling her out of the operating room, she sensed herself return to her real body again. In the following days, she told her parents about what she had felt and heard and the doctors confirmed what had been said. Describing the events, both women wanted me to understand how remarkable the experience had been; neither had been terribly upset by it.

With the patient 'asleep', 'relaxed' and pain-free, maintaining stability is also the duty of the anaesthetist – a task like keeping pulse rate, blood pressure and oxygen levels steady while car-crash-scale assault is taking place on a person's chest. They need a reliable drip to give access to the patient's circulation to administer drugs or blood. In the early days it was the job of the surgical team with their scalpels to cut down through the skin on to a big vein and insert a fat metal needle in the arm or ankle, secure it with bandages and a splint and hook it up through some red-rubber tubing to a hanging glass bottle full of clear liquid; these incisions add to the high scar counts of many of the early patients. Currently anaesthetists insert one or more soft plastic tubes into the veins of the neck, hooked up via clear plastic tubing to floppy plastic bags of fluid.

Compared to Lorraine's 1938 first ductus operation, settling the patient on the operating table takes longer now that there are so many monitoring wires to connect. At some stage, the anaesthetist sets up a bar above the patient's neck demarcating one side as the surgeon's territory, the other side as the anaesthetist's; one side is kept sterile, the other merely clean: the 'blood-brain barrier' (anaesthetist's joke). Before continuous monitoring of oxygen levels became possible, some anaesthetists draped their side of the bar with white drapes, the better to gauge the colour of the child's lips.

While Lorraine's nurse simply tried to keep a finger free to check the child's pulse, the monitoring lines attached to a modern patient include ECG wires to monitor heart rate and rhythm, and a pulse oximeter to continuously read their oxygen saturations. Screens show wiggly lines displaying the levels of the various gases going in and out of the patient and document breath-by-breath how stiff the lungs are. Temperature is followed both on the skin and also somewhere deep in the body, blood pressure is typically tracked using a tube in an artery at the wrist and the pressure in a central vein from another in a neck vein. A nerve stimulator checks whether the child is sufficiently 'relaxed' (muscles paralysed), an echo probe sited in the gullet offers a view of the heart's plumbing and function from behind, and some units use NIRS (near-infrared spectroscopy: a trendy technology that measures the oxygen content of brain tissue; the aim is to reduce the chance of brain damage on bypass). Regular checks of the oxygen and acid levels in the blood and of clotting function are available using what we now call 'near-patient' technology. Then there is the job of keeping track of all the blood and other fluids going in and out of the patient and all the drugs involved in keeping the child safe and asleep. While the surgeon concentrates on what is going on in the hole in the chest, it is the anaesthetist who holds the 'situational awareness'.

The cast-list for Lorraine's operation in 1938 was small: two surgeons and a nurse were scrubbed-up and another nurse managed the anaesthetic; spectators watched from a viewing gallery. Fifteen years later, a visitor watching the early cross-circulation operations like Mickey Shaw's in the early 1950s thought the operating room was 'like a circus', so many performers, so much to-ing and fro-ing. The cast-list for current operations has shrunk again. Surgeons all now wear headlights, much like a miner's; many incorporate cameras hooked up to remote screens so that a trainee can get a 'surgeon's eye view' from outside the operating room. This leaves two or three surgeons, an anaesthetist perhaps with a helper, a scrubbed nurse and one or two people driving the machinery that takes over the job of the heart. There are screens everywhere and a lot of alarms.

The Dome in London was first built for the new millennium as an extravagant exhibition space. One of the experiences offered was a walkthrough of a 'hospital of the future'. In the operating room, there was only one human being: the patient. The surgeon was outside drinking coffee. He was wearing virtual-reality goggles to remotely control a robot that was doing the bloody work. The anaesthetist was sitting at a bank of computer screens responsible for administering several different anaesthetics simultaneously. This scenario may well be coming.

★　★　★

I am in awe of what cardiac anaesthetists do – an anaesthetic mis-judgement can certainly kill a patient more quickly than a surgical one – so I am curious about why the patients and parents I talked to seemed so blasé about anaesthesia. They seem ready to talk about the thirty seconds that it takes to put a child to sleep but then take for granted the following hours when the anaesthetist is their child's guardian angel. On reflection, I suspect that during their child's operation they simply had no emotional space for any more worry.

Everyone enters the operating room determined. For every heart operation, there is a moment when the professional team becomes committed to its success. This occurs long beforehand at a meeting where each patient's story and their diagnostic information are individually reviewed; there may be thirty people in the room – cardiologists, anaesthetists, surgeons, nurses and trainees. The options and timings of what to do for the best are debated, and when the discussion wraps up, a cardiologist and a surgeon will record and sign off the conclusion. After that, there are no further reservations – the whole team will see the decision through to the end. Some time later, a corresponding conversation happens between the surgeon and the patient or their family, pictures are sketched and competence hopefully conveyed. More paperwork is signed and seals the complete sense of commitment. After these signatures, hesitation is out of place and all anyone wants to talk about is hope.

9
Cold hearts

Warren Mauston had one of the first ever pacemakers in 1959 – without it, he had no pulse at all. A wire sewn onto his heart came out through his skin and was attached to a 'pulse generator' box that he carried around with him. Later, when miniaturization allowed pulse generators to be implanted under the skin, he declined (his explanation being that his grandmother had refused indoor plumbing because 'some things just don't belong inside'). He came to enjoy a certain cachet as a celebrity patient, willing to demonstrate the technology to visiting doctors. His surgeon explains:

> He allowed me . . . to turn off the pacemaker and time how long before he slipped into unconsciousness . . . If I set him at 60 [beats per minute] and then turned [it] off – bang – he would be OK for four beats. For four seconds. And then he would start to slide and go unconscious or begin to twitch. And he always said he was falling back, sort of down a well or down a big barrel. And he said it wasn't unpleasant. Then I'd snap it on again, and he'd come right out of it.

If your heart simply stops, you lose consciousness quickly. At about forty seconds, your pupils dilate – the tell-tale sign that brain activity has stopped. Breathing stops. After that, all tissues in the body survive for a while – how long varies from tissue to tissue, even cell-type to cell-type. For example, compared to arm-muscle cells, heart-muscle cells are very vulnerable. But the brain is the most susceptible of all tissues to being deprived of blood. If effective circulation is somehow restored within about three minutes, there is a good chance that the brain will recover completely, but beyond that time the injury is not reversible, even if normal blood flow is restored. This means that, without some sort of 'damage limitation' strategy to protect the brain, three minutes is the longest time a heart can be stopped.

For most of the first three decades of the development of open-heart surgery, the operational definition of death revolved around the notion of the heart stopping. Yet to complete an open-heart operation, the surgeon needs literally to stop the heart, open it up to the air and peek inside (and needs to do this for longer than three minutes). So does this mean that the patient has been dead? The evolution of heart surgery has taught that, if the conditions are right, hearts that have stopped may be restarted, bodies that have been cold and stiff one day may be sitting up in bed the next, and people may even walk out of hospital without a heartbeat – as do patients with modern 'artificial hearts', which often circulate the blood continuously rather than by reproducing a pulse. To retain any connotation of irreversibility or finality, the legal designation of 'death' has had to morph over the decades since cardiac surgery came into being* and now most practical definitions revolve around the concept of 'brain death'.

---

* Breaching legal definitions has not perturbed cardiac surgeons much, but law-makers continue to struggle. For many years in the USA, in principle somebody could be 'brought back to life' by crossing the border between two adjacent states that had different definitions of the point of death.

Many cultures have aspired to bring people back from the dead. The 'Amsterdam Society for the Recovery of Drowned Persons' founded in 1767 was the first to try methods that were plausible to modern understanding (tip water out of the lungs, don't despair too soon) – but it took almost two centuries before resuscitation became a project for truly investigatory medical science. In the 1920s at the Johns Hopkins Hospital in Baltimore, surgeons gave their own anaesthetics; the speciality of anaesthesia had not emerged. If a patient stopped breathing during an operation, it was the hospital's fire department that was called. They would rush in to press the masks of their 'powered respirators' to blow oxygen on to the patient's face.

Even during the 1940s and 1950s when congenital heart surgery was beginning, if a patient's heart stopped on the ward after an operation, their breathing would stop moments later and everyone would watch helplessly as the child died before their eyes. If the child was in the vicinity of an operating room, the surgical team might rush to cut open their chest and squeeze the heart from within to try to maintain some circulation and possibly reverse whatever downward spiral had caused the cardiac arrest. But this devastating trauma was almost always unsuccessful.*

At this point, 'rescue breathing' (puffing into the victim's mouth) was believed to be ineffective and the 'closed chest cardiac massage' we see on TV had still not been invented. The benefit of artificial respiration by mouth-to-mouth breathing was not proven until the mid 1950s. The clinching demonstration involved thirty-one volunteer medical students and doctors

---

* Dr Paul Wood, the most inspirational British cardiologist of his era, knew the futility of such theatricals. When he diagnosed the 'irreversibility' of his own heart attack, he made his team promise that they would not let anyone open his chest. Later when he collapsed, they watched silently as his ECG deteriorated and he died in 1962.

who agreed* to be paralysed with drugs that rendered them completely unable to breathe for themselves. They were then 'breathed' mouth-to-mouth, first by the instructing anaesthetist and then by any of the fire-fighters, policemen, soldiers, Boy Scouts, housewives or other spectators who wanted to have a go.

Even if rescuers could get oxygen in and out of the lungs, they still needed a way of getting the blood to circulate around the body. During an experiment on a dog, someone had noticed that pressing hard on its chest after its heart had stopped produced a discernible pulse in its neck. Occasional reports of resuscitation of humans by pumping on their chests began to appear in medical journals in the late 1950s. By the early 1960s, mouth-to-mouth breathing and chest compressions had been brought together as Cardio-Pulmonary Resuscitation (CPR) in a 'package' that could be taught to medical staff and later to lay people.[†] A woman who was a London nurse in the 1950s and 1960s remembers how enthusiastically staff embraced their new brief, which was to attempt to resuscitate every patient who was showing signs of dying in hospital. The victims would often be dragged off the bed and on to the floor, the better to pump hard on their chests. Though screens would be pulled around the drama, other patients could not possibly avoid knowing what was happening.

Patrick was carried into his Manchester hospital when he was four years old and by 1964 he was five, able to walk and a veteran of the ward. He remembers slipping away from the other children who were being shepherded towards the playroom as the screens were swished around a bed. He peeped through the curtain to watch,

---

* They did agree – though they were also paid $150 for each stint (a resident's monthly pay at the time was about $100).

† The first mannequin made for learners to practice on was 'Miss Sweet Breath'. She was the ancestor of the more convincing 'Resusci Annie' which is still used, originally made by a Norwegian toymaker.

fascinated, as a crowd of doctors and nurses failed to resuscitate a boy called Tommy. 'Cold with fear and excitement', he continued to observe as the nurses cried, Tommy's parents cried, and Tommy was wrapped in a sheet and put into a 'silver bullet on wheels' to be trundled away by Fred and Mike, the hospital porters. The following morning he asked Sister Mann if everybody left in a trolley like that. Patrick, now a priest in his fifties, has seen more than his share of death, but this encounter when he was five was his first.

★   ★   ★

But what of those three minutes before the brain starts to die? The first great challenge of open-heart surgery was to take control of that time and so extend it. Over the years, there have been four strategies for dealing with the brain's vulnerability to lack of oxygen while a heart is open and not producing any circulation: speed, cooling, cross-circulation and heart-lung machines.

The first strategy was for surgeons to choose a very simple problem and work really, really fast. Three minutes is not long. To even see what they are doing, the surgeon must open the heart and suck the blood out, find the defect, place their stitches and close the heart – all in the time it takes you to brush your teeth. On the plus side, speed had always been at a premium in surgery, a legacy from the time when amputations were done without anaesthesia. But realistically there is a very limited choice of problems inside the heart that can be dealt with in three minutes – perhaps a straight-forward hole between the collecting chambers, closing an Atrial Septal Defect (ASD).

Even in the new millennium, closing an ASD is still done in this speedy 'smash and grab' style somewhere in the world. In 2014, an Iranian group reported closing simple ASDs without a heart-lung machine. They opened each patient's chest, temporarily stopped blood from getting into the heart (by compressing the veins as they entered from the upper and lower body), cut through the wall of the right atrium, sucked the blood out of the cavity, exposed the hole between the atria, closed the ASD with two quick rows of sutures, released the veins, allowed the heart to fill again and closed their entry hole. Their longest time inside any of 130 hearts repaired in this way was eighty seconds.

This Iranian team was using modern surgical instruments and could be confident of the diagnosis; they even had a machine standing by, ready to take over the patient's heart and lung function if needed. But this was not the case at the beginning of open-heart surgery – the surgeons' equipment and lighting were primitive by present standards, they had to confirm the diagnosis (which was not always correct) and there was no Plan B.

For more extensive operations, the early surgeons needed a little more time, so capitalized on the knowledge that at lower temperatures cells die more slowly. The first successful open-heart operation was done in Minnesota in 1952 when a five-year-old child called Jacqueline was anaesthetized and wrapped in a 'refrigeration blanket'. When her temperature reached 28°C (normal is 37°C) her chest was opened and the operation completed in the same way as the Iranians have done more recently. Once her chest was closed, she was put in a bath filled with hot water, rewarmed, wiped down and returned to the ward. Her heart had been emptied and her circulation stopped for five minutes and the hypothermia had protected her brain cells.* In 1958 Ben Milstein, a surgeon at Papworth Hospital in England, performed their first open-heart operation, another ASD repair. The surgery went well and at the end of the operation the elated team seized the surgeon and threw him into the ice-bath. Mr Milstein records 'they had very decently emptied it and refilled it with warm water'.

In the early 1960s the British were still relying on cooling techniques to protect their patients' brains as the operating times

---

* Dr Lillehei, Mickey Shaw's surgeon, assisted at this operation.

extended, but they were removing the baths from their operating suites. Ice baths had always been a bit of an emotional challenge for staff as well as patients. The early pictures of naked patients lying anaesthetized in roll-top domestic baths, their heads lolling where the taps might be, were reminiscent of the mental images of concentration camp prisoners conjured up during the Nuremberg trials of the Nazi doctors. (In Dachau, internees were plunged into freezing water, dressed in aviators' uniforms but fully conscious and begging their 'doctors' to be hauled out.)*

For a patient whose heart was to be exposed anyway, it seemed more aesthetically pleasing and practical to cool their blood rather than their skin. This needed an 'extracorporeal' circuit. By the end of the 1940s, kidney doctors had already sorted out how to put tubes into the blood vessels of their patients with renal failure, stop the blood clotting in the pipes,† pump it out to a machine which 'dialysed' it and return the 'improved' blood into the patient's circulation.‡ In the same way, the 1950s cardiac surgeons simply bought pumps from catalogues and used them to move blood around. The Minnesota team's pumps came from the dairy industry, the Great Ormond Street team used

* The Nuremberg Doctors' Trial got underway in 1946 and a Polish Catholic priest who had survived gave testimony. The ice bath experiments were ostensibly conducted to learn how best to rewarm airmen who had ditched into the sea. The subsequent use of this data for informing clinical hypothermia for heart surgery was contested, because of the coercion the Nazi experiments had entailed.
† The substance that came to be called heparin was first isolated from dog liver by a medical student at Johns Hopkins in 1916; it anti-coagulates the blood. Its effects are reversed by protamine, discovered in 1874 in salmon sperm.
‡ Dialysis substitutes for kidney function by removing urea and other food by-products from the blood. The first successful 'haemodialysis' for kidney failure was in 1945. (On waking from her uremic coma, the woman's first words were 'I'm going to divorce my husband.')

roller-pumps from the Chivers jam factory (the pumps were gentle enough to avoid over-squishing the strawberries). The team could open the patient's chest, put some tubes into the veins coming into the heart and divert the blood through some outside-the-body cooling apparatus before returning it to the heart which then circulated the cold blood around the whole body. The brain was protected by this 'hypothermia', and with this 'extracorporeal' technology a new team of operating-room helpers was born – the 'perfusionists' who controlled the pumps and cooling apparatus.

With their patients cooled to around 30°C, the surgeons had about ten minutes' operating time before brain damage was inevitable. This permitted some slightly more complicated operations, including work on the pulmonary and aortic valves. But if a surgeon was to rely on 'hypothermia' alone, the cooling had to be taken a whole lot lower than 30°C to gain enough time for more complicated problems inside the heart to be tackled. At the Westminster Hospital in London, the chief surgeon co-opted a refrigeration engineer who had made equipment for ice-cream factories.* His apparatus for 'profound hypothermia' was made in the hospital workshop in around 1960 and is now held at the London Science Museum.† His exact remit was to build equipment that would take a body weighing 150 pounds down from 37°C to 15°C in half an hour and then back up again to 37°C, with an extracorporeal blood flow of three litres per minute, the blood temperature never falling below 4°C nor rising above 40°C.

---

* This was David Shore who worked for APV, the company later responsible for the tour de force of manufacturing the Cadbury's Creme Egg. How do they do that?

† Richard, who had survived surgery in the 1970s, was thirty in 1994 when he visited the London Science Museum where this machine was displayed – he remembers it as massive.

The anaesthetist would ventilate the patient's lungs throughout the cooling time. The machinery had pneumatic controls and separate refrigeration and heating units and was so large that it did not fit in the operating theatre and was set up in a corridor or in an adjacent room.

Once the patient was cooled below 15°C, all the machinery was simply turned off and no blood circulated. The cold heart had long stopped beating, the lungs were rested and the anaesthetist went for a coffee break – 'circulatory arrest' meant that it was pointless even to give drugs. The 'deep hypothermia and circulatory arrest' seemed to permit the surgeon to operate at some leisure on a still, cold, empty heart. Seeing one body's temperature down at 8°C, a visiting surgeon remarked that the patient was 'pretty damn cold' – but the evidence at the time suggested that the brain was safe with no circulation for an hour at that temperature. Controlling the machinery was a nightmare for both anaesthetist and perfusionists, since two pumps were required (one to pump blood round the body and the other to pump blood round the lungs). Keeping the two pump outputs synchronized required enormous skill and attention and no small amount of luck. However, the surgeon was happy – and he was the 'captain of the ship'.

Susan's heart was repaired using this machine in 1961. She was nine years old and remembers being one of ten children operated on during the visit of a US surgeon – and one of only three who survived. Postoperatively she left her sheltered school that had low academic aspirations to compete with her 'run of the mill' contemporaries. Many years later she got a first-class degree in education, so her brain cannot have been too damaged during the long time when she had no circulation at all. And her heart repair has since served her through two pregnancies.

The alternative to hypothermia that the Minnesota team used in 1954 to repair Mickey Shaw's heart was 'cross-circulation'. All

they needed was a donor and a pump that could accurately control
the blood passing backwards and forwards between the two bodies.
The donor's lungs provided the oxygen for both bodies (and the
donor's liver almost certainly helped minimize the amount of acid
that would build up in the child's body because the rate of circulation provided by the pump was never quite enough). No other
unit is ever recorded as using this technique and as soon as they
had developed a reliable heart-lung machine, the Minnesota team
abandoned the use of donors.*

From the early 1950s, several US and Canadian centres had
started building prototype machines to take over the work of both
the heart and lungs. If they could be perfected, these would do
away with the intense time pressures that surgeons had to work
under – and more complicated heart problems could be tackled.
There was a lot to understand, but the gung-ho and somewhat
competitive and secretive atmosphere prevented teams learning
from each other. The contenders in the contest for status were
self-taught, their experimental work was done on dogs, cats and
pigs, and progress was largely due to trial and error. Moving the
blood around (mimicking the work of the heart) was quickly
achieved, but oxygenating it (mimicking the work of the lungs
without smashing up the blood cells) was a real difficulty. The
very first successful open-heart operation using a heart-lung
machine incorporating an 'oxygenator' was in 1953 in Jefferson
Medical College, Philadelphia. By 1955, eighteen patients had been

---

* Pam, another survivor I talked to, was supported during her operation by
her father. She became another 'poster girl' for the programme – and a 'daddy's
girl' through her childhood (she wasn't told of his part in her operation until
afterwards). But it is her mother that she felt for – on the 'worst day of her life',
her mother could have lost her two most precious people.

operated using different mechanical 'heart-lung machines' in six different centres and only one had survived.*

It took years for these machines to be built commercially, but by the mid 1950s US medical teams were turning to industry for help; suddenly heart surgery seemed worth investing in. In the USA, International Business Machines (IBM) and General Motors got stuck in alongside their respective clinical teams (at the Mayo Clinic and in Detroit), starting a competitive race and building heart-lung machines that were said to resemble office equipment (specifically punch-card sorters) and car engines (specifically Cadillac engines) respectively. In the UK, despite the government medical research agency declining to bankroll the development of a British prototype and venture capital funding being scarce, a machine was built and first used on patients in the Hammersmith Hospital, London in 1957. It worked fairly consistently, but took a couple of working days to clean between runs. For the next five years British units were still working on a shoestring – the Papworth team used the Hammersmith equipment to practise on pigs in a gardener's hut in the grounds of the Cambridge Veterinary School, wearing ski-suits under their gowns because the space was so cold.

Even when it was human beings having real operations while relying on the early machines, surgeons needed to be ready to improvise. A surgeon from San Francisco tells the story of their oxygenator of the time:

---

* The estimate of the number of deaths is an 'at least' number – it is very likely that some failures were not documented. Five of the eighteen reported operations used monkey lungs and one used a human lung excised at post-mortem as the oxygenator. The rest got oxygen into the blood by passing a film of it across a membrane or passing bubbles through the blood while it was in the extracorporeal circuit.

It was a series of plastic bags, on the inside of which venous [blue] blood was sprayed with the help of a Chevrolet windshield wiper. Periodically there would be a sound of breaking glass and a muttered 'damn' with dusky blood – because it wasn't a very good oxygenator – spreading around our boots. [The surgeon] never even blinked as he continued quietly closing the defect. This taught me an important lesson; that it is seldom the first mistake that leads to death on the operating table. It is so commonly a second mistake made by a member of the team under pressure from the first.

Another doctor, from Papworth, described how the equipment was working fine

> until suddenly the heat exchanger – a brass connection on it – gave way and I felt blood running down my back and I looked round and I saw . . . air going [down] the tube towards the patient so I quickly clamped it [to] stop . . . air going in, and reverted the patient to [her] own circulation. [The staff] dismantled the equipment, [and sent it] by a very fast car, with a police escort, to the Engineering School, who repaired the brazing of the connection on the heat exchanger, came back to Papworth with it, sterilized it, the patient was still asleep, the operation continued and the patient didn't know what had happened!

These days the components of a heart-lung machine are bought from commercial companies and many parts are disposable. Typically open-heart surgery now leaves the patient dependent on a heart-lung machine (a.k.a. 'on pump' or 'on bypass') for as long as the surgeon needs to be inside the heart. The blood – and hence the body – is still usually cooled a little so that the surgeon can temporarily drop the flow rates in the circuit if blood starts to obscure his field of view. A child having Fallot's tetralogy repaired could be 'on bypass' for three hours.

Then there is usually a moment of apprehension when the main job is done and it is time for the repaired heart to take over again from the machine. (In my first cardiac surgical job, Rossini's *William Tell* overture would be turned on at this moment.) There is a lot less tension and shouting in operating rooms nowadays, but various things can still go wrong. The heart may stay completely unresponsive – still as a stone. Or it may wriggle but not beat. Or it may beat, but terribly slowly. Finally, it may just not work very well.

These problems correspond to damage that hearts can sustain while on bypass. Normal heart muscle wants to beat – it has an intrinsic rhythm, a propensity to pump. If a healthy heart is full of blood it beats strongly, and even if it is empty it will still pulsate a little. Thus, when the main operation is over, it may be enough to simply let the heart fill up with blood and wait for the natural coordinated pumping to resume. Because so many lessons have been learned over the years, this is what happens after almost every operation now. But historically this could not be taken for granted, especially if the surgeon had needed to deliberately stop the heart beating.

For a simple operation like closing an atrial hole, the stitching did not have to be too precise and some inherent pulsation of the heart was not too inconvenient. But for more ambitious operations where stitches needed to be accurately placed a millimetre apart, a moving target became a real problem. Finding a way of stopping any pulsation became vital. One option was simply to deprive the heart of oxygen by blocking blood flow down the coronary arteries that feed the heart muscle itself; without oxygen the heart beats itself to a standstill. Unfortunately a sort of 'rigor mortis' of the heart often follows and these 'stone hearts' proved very difficult to restart. If it is impossible to wean the circulation from the heart-lung machine, the patient will die on the operating table. A better method of stopping the heart while protecting its muscle emerged in the late 1950s. Running a potassium solution down the heart's own arteries turned off contractions like a sort of chemical switch; if the solution was also very cold, the heart muscle would be better preserved too. Variants of this technique are used to the present day and 'stone hearts' are very rare.

The second feared scenario when weaning from the heart-lung machine was ventricular fibrillation (VF). Each unit of muscle squirms at its own rate with no overall synchronicity. In the very early days, before anything could be done about it, this was distressing to see – the muscle seemed to work but was unable to get its act together to pump in a coordinated way.

The trick doctors learned to deal with VF used electricity. In the early 1900s, after several operatives had died by accidental electrocution, the General Electric Company commissioned some research into what made electric shocks lethal. One experimental team was shocking stray dogs to death and noticed that sometimes a second shock would revive them. Researchers started tinkering and by 1947 the first successful resuscitation was achieved when a fourteen-year-old boy lived after being defibrillated ('shocked') after he went into VF during an operation on his ribs. Making the equipment mobile was the next challenge. By 1965, defibrillators could be fired from an ambulance's starter battery and now the units we see on train stations and in other public places can 'read' the victim's heart rhythm and automatically deliver the correct size of shock if a brave member of the public takes the initiative to help. The most 'intelligent' defibrillators are now fully implantable into people whose heart rhythms repeatedly misbehave; they are small but deliver a kick which some patients will tell us about later.

The third situation that early surgeons dreaded was seeing the

heart take over after an operation but with a very slow heartbeat. 'Heart block' was one of the main killers in Lillehei's early
cross-circulation operations. The intrinsic rhythm of heart muscle
is rather slow, but there is an area at the top of the right atrium
that naturally beats faster. The heart has a specialized 'conducting
system' that allows this little area to act as the 'pacemaker' of the
normal heart and coordinates its supple and synchronized pumping. Crucially, the conducting system includes a 'relay' situated
in the middle of the heart through which the beat is conducted
onwards through the ventricular muscle by bundles of 'cables'.
Unfortunately it took some children's deaths before the surgeons
realized that some of the stitches they were inserting to close
Ventricular Septal Defects (VSDs) were going right through the
relay node. If the electrical connection between the natural pacemaker at the top of the atria is blocked from reaching the main
pumping muscle, the ventricles revert to their slow intrinsic rate,
which is just too slow to keep the body going. The children would
get back to the ward and slowly fade and die. A few adults had
been tided over temporary 'heart block' by the firing of regular
50–150-volt electrical shocks through electrodes strapped to their
chests, but this was torture for children, who would tear off the
contraption.

The urgent task of keeping the heart going artificially was
solved in the garages of Minneapolis by the predecessors of the
now massive Medtronic medical device company. Their first pacemaker was powered from the mains and delivered small regular
beats directly to 'blocked' hearts via a wire loosely sewn onto the
surface of the heart muscle; 1.5 volts was sufficient to ensure pacing
and the children could not feel the shocks. With this arrangement,
paced children could not move far from a wall-plug – they could
not even be moved from the operating room to the ward in a lift.
After a child died during a power cut, a battery-operated system
was conceived. This was devised and first tried out in a dog and

then, the very next day, on a post-operative little girl.* The first
internal pacemaker was implanted in Sweden in 1958. One end of
the wire was stitched onto the outside of the patient's heart and the
other end was tunnelled towards a battery encapsulated in a mould
made from a shoe-polish tin and sewn under the patient's abdominal skin. Five lead-systems, twenty-two batteries and forty-two
years later, that patient died at the age of eighty-four.

Finally, a repaired heart may struggle off-bypass beating unhap-
pily, swelling up or not emptying properly. While it is possible to
go 'back on pump' for a while, this cannot be sustained indefinitely.
If the team is sure that the repair cannot be improved upon, a 'sink
or swim' time has to come sooner or later. A child's death on the
operating table has become a very rare event, mainly due to the
innumerable small improvements in diagnosis, surgical planning
and advances in drugs and bypass technology. But there is now
also one more card to play: with modified pumps and oxygenators,
bypass can be extended if necessary for days. This Extracorporeal
Life Support (ECLS) is very rarely used, but has saved occasional
patients whose hearts or lungs or both have needed long recovery
times. The first child who was saved by this technology in the
aftermath of a congenital heart operation had had a Mustard repair
(see page 277) for Transposition of the Great Arteries in California
in 1972; for about twenty hours the circuit provided complete rest
for his heart and lungs before the equipment was gradually, then
completely, turned off after thirty-four hours.

---

* This is the story always quoted to support the 'ready, fire, aim' era of medical technology development. One writer who studied Medtronic noted: 'The
garage . . . symbolized an unfettered state where technical genius and creativ-
ity could be applied for the betterment of mankind.' By 1976, the FDA did
not agree. Because so many problems only emerged after a device had been
implanted resulted in product recalls and in the light of shady marketing prac-
tices, they stepped in to insist on extensive testing before devices were implanted
into humans.

ECLS is a treatment of last resort now, and only used in situations that *both* seem unsurvivable if nothing is done *and* where there is some realistic hope that time will heal whatever problem has brought the child to such a parlous state. Whether it is just the heart that is being substituted (by a Ventricular Assist Device (VAD))* or the lungs (Extracorporeal Membrane Oxygenation (ECMO)) or both, the equipment is extensive, scary and brings problems of its own. It is hard for a parent — or anyone who is unprepared for the sight — to see a child's blood snaking through tubing, pumps and reservoirs, the child himself lying improbably still, not even breathing and with a face swollen, waxen and often unrecognizable. ECLS is brutal to the body. Malfunction of some component of the equipment or a clot in the tubing can happen at any moment, so each time a parent kisses a hand or a foot before leaving the room for a break they know that this might be a goodbye kiss. The stress goes on for days, but sooner or later the make-or-break moment arrives. Some hearts recover and the children stabilize, but ECLS is a life-saving treatment that does not save every life. Sometimes we ask medicine to do more than it can.

---

* These are the 'artificial hearts' that are currently used to keep deteriorating patients alive while waiting for a heart transplant — but completely synthetic implantable hearts are a holy grail for cardiologists, patients and commercial manufacturers.

10

'It's a very detailed and complex operation . . .'*

How to repair tetralogy of Fallot†(don't try this at home)

Wearing your mask, hat and scrubs, headlight and magnifying-loupes, choose your gloves from the rack: glove sizes 5½ for the most minuscule scrub nurse to 8½ for the most magnificent surgeon. Peel open the packet and carefully drop the insert containing your gloves folded in a wrap of crisp paper down beside the paper towel on the trolley carrying your sterile gown.

Move to the long stainless-steel trough that acts as a communal basin to scrub. Using your elbows, turn on the taps and organize the water to a comfortable temperature. Open a new nailbrush packet and, again with your elbow, squirt a generous dose of brown (iodine) or pink (a liquid likely to have 'x' in its name) onto the

---

* 'It's a very detailed and complex operation' was said to a mother by her child's surgeon. Patronizing or realistic? You decide.

† Reminder of the 'tetralogy' components: 1. there is a large hole between the two pumping chambers (VSD); 2. the aorta sits directly above this hole it 'overrides'; 3. there is some blockage between the right ventricle and the lung artery; and 4. the wall of the right ventricle is unusually thick.

brush. Off you go, squirting, brushing and rinsing for ten full minutes. If others are scrubbing, small-talk is usual. Up to the elbows,
pay particular attention to your fingernails.*

That done, clasp your dripping hands as if in prayer and
approach the gown trolley. Pick up the paper towel without touching anything else and dry your hands completely, throwing the
towel into a non-sterile bin. Put on your surgical gown. Made of
paper or cotton, it is like a coat worn back to front and will have
been folded so that you need only touch its inside. Arms go in first,
then hoist the gown over the front of your body and shrug it over
your shoulders. Keep your hands inside the sleeves. Try to look
nonchalant; someone else will be fastening the ties at the back.

Attend now to the gloves. Flick the folded paper package open.
You will see that the gloves are arranged left glove on the left, right
glove on the right with about three inches of cuff being folded
up towards the fingers to help you dive your hand in. Using the
sleeved 'stump' of your gown-covered right hand, lift the left glove
off the trolley by hooking into the fold between the fingers and its
cuff. Wriggle your left hand out of its sleeve and into the interior
of the glove. This is a clumsy motion for several reasons; there will
be wrinkles and misplaced fingers inside this left glove, but don't
worry. Now with the left glove awkwardly on, use it to lift the right
glove off its paper and similarly onto your right hand. (If you are
sufficiently important a nurse may help you with all this.) Now there
is a delicious moment of pinging and snapping as you work all your
fingers properly into their rubbery skin. If a residual wrinkle snags on
a needle, you will need to ask for a new pair of gloves in the middle
of some drama. Arrange the gloves to cover the cuffs of your gown.

Approach the operating table where the patient is lying, the
anaesthetist's paraphernalia in place. With anaesthetist, scrub nurse

---

* Instructors of the past covered the trainees' forearms in sooty oil and blind-
folded them while they scrubbed.

and perfusionists present, confirm that you all agree who the patient is and what operation is to be performed; this is not the first time this has been checked, but it will be the last. Draw a line on the skin where you anticipate making your incision. Stand back while the scrub nurse paints the patient's chest with brown Betadine sterilizing swabs and waits for it to dry. You may help place a clear sticky film to cover the middle of the patient's chest. Drape the rest of their torso with whatever drapes you are offered; they will probably be made of waxy paper. Receive from the perfusionists the sterile ends of the clear tubing that will later connect the child to the heart-lung machine. They are full of fluid and have their ends clamped; secure them to the drapes, level with your midriff. As the surgical team clusters around the table and the field of view diminishes, everyone's focus changes. To create a 'moment', perhaps ask the anaesthetist: 'Ready to start?'

Use a scalpel to incise the skin; just stroke along your mark, no need to press hard; a bright red line appears. Use a diathermy tool to cut deeper and to burn and seal small bleeders; be careful, it's hot. With your fingers in the uppermost part of the wound, find the top of the breastbone and the inter-clavicular ligament joining the collarbones; divide it with your diathermy. (If the names of structures are not familiar, don't worry; the doing of surgery has little to do with language.) There is a vein up there that frequently bleeds and another at the bottom of the breastbone – the 'Veins of Sod'; control them and when everything is dry, score the front of the sternum with your diathermy.

To open the chest, accept the saw the scrub nurse offers you. This will probably be a sophisticated oscillating saw that you use to cut downwards onto and through the sternum; needless to say, the breastbone of a child is soft; use your judgement. Apply some wax to seal the exposed sternal marrow and use the diathermy to curtail any new bleeding. Slip the two blades of the metal retractor under the two cut halves of the sternum; these will come to frame your view of the heart as you work. Wind the blades of the retractor apart to crank the chest open; this may feel a bit brutal. In front of you is the thymus. You will need to remove most of it; it has a capsule allowing it to be gently peeled away, uncovering a vein beneath. You will be able to open the retractor a little more and expose the pericardium – the sac that surrounds the heart.

Incise the pericardium vertically using the diathermy and open it as you would double doors, revealing the heart inside; keep the 'doors' open with strong sutures attaching to the pericardium and lay more drapes to keep your working area clear of clutter. The heart of a child is about the size of his own fist; Fallot repairs are generally done before the age of one; go figure. The heart glistens, the colour of veal. It is beating comfortably. Don't touch it yet.

The next stage is to get in some tubes so that you can safely empty the heart. Call for heparin to be given so that the blood will not clot in the tubes. The 'venous' pipes you insert will drain off the blue blood as it arrives back into the heart and divert it to the heart-lung machine. The machine will oxygenate it and then return the bright-red blood through an 'arterial' tube that you will place in the aorta – and will deliver the blood under enough pressure to send it around the body. This arrangement bypasses the heart and lungs, the body gets the oxygen and blood flow it needs and you can open the heart.

First find the two major veins as they enter the bottom and top of the right atrium and free them up from their surrounding tissues – tubes will later go into each to drain blue blood out. Attend to the aorta which is immediately in front of you as it leaves the heart. Put two careful concentric circular 'purse string' sutures into the aorta's wall – when you pull on these, they will snug down on the cannula you will insert into the patient's aorta. Put similar purse strings near where each of the big veins enters the heart and a third on the ear-shaped appendage on the front of the right atrium. As you prepare to cannulate the aorta, you will notice your 'intention-tremor' magnified in your spectacle-loupes. Steady yourself as you accept a pointy scalpel. Focus on the spot in the middle of the aortic purse string. Stab into the aorta – far enough but not too far. This is an anxious moment – keep your eyes on the spot. Between you and your assistant opposite, nudge the plastic aortic cannula so that its tip is inside the aorta itself and immediately snug the purse-string around the cannula to control the high-pressure bleeding. Join up this aortic cannula to the correct section of tubing that you have been nursing under your tummy. So far, you have avoided touching the heart itself – just as well because it is still doing all the pump-work. But now you need to establish connections to drain blood from the body to the machine. To get on bypass, it's probably safest to put your first cannula through the middle of the purse-string around the handy ear-like appendage in the front of the atrium; manoeuvres there do not require too much poking of the beating heart. Then, avoiding letting air into the tubes, join the heart-end and the machine-ends of the venous tubings together and you are ready to go.

With a pipe in the aorta and another in the atrium and everyone calm, you can let the heart-lung machine start to do the work. From now, you can entrust control of the circulation to the perfusionists and anaesthetists who will maintain correct pressures, monitor the patient's clotting, oxygenation and temperature from their respective 'flight decks'. They will stop ventilating the lungs. They will cool the blood and hence the patient's body and brain. You can handle the heart with impunity now – but until the atrial cannula is moved, you can't open the atrium. Separately cannulate the large veins as they enter the right atrium using the purse-strings you placed earlier and tighten tapes around both veins so that all the blood is diverted into the machine and none reaches the heart.

You are not yet quite ready to open the heart: the heart is still beating and there is still some blood pooling inside. It has come down the coronary arteries, supplied the heart muscle and returned to the right atrium; even this coronary blood flow needs to be cut off if you are to be able to see where to put your stitches. You will see where the coronary arteries come off the aorta, just as it leaves the heart. There is enough space to put a clamp above the coronaries but below the aortic cannula and so interrupt the heart's own blood supply. But now the heart muscle needs protection from lack of oxygen, so insert a little cannula between the heart and the clamp and infuse some cold potassium solution into it; this will immediately stop and relax the heart.

You may now cut open the right atrium and suck out the blood and potassium solution that will be sloshing around inside it. This incision will be your window into the heart, so you will need to keep it held open. Use the handy ridge of muscle inside the atrium to place some stay-sutures and lay open the atrium; you will be able to see the tricuspid valve at the base of the chamber. To avoid cutting the heart's valuable pumping muscle, you will need to do all your work on the Ventricular Septal Defect (VSD) and on the blocked outflow tract through this valve; its circumference in an infant is about the size of a big man's wedding ring, though more pliable. Place some suction tubes; you want the inside of the heart to be dry.

Now you can rummage around and assess the anatomy. Your assistant can help you get a decent look at the VSD if they gently retract the tricuspid valve; you will have to stoop and peer upwards to get a good view. Check that you know exactly where the nearby aortic valve is (you don't want to snag that in a stitch) and the conducting system (ditto). Have a preliminary look at the way out from right ventricle to pulmonary artery; you can use your finger to assess the too-bulky muscle that is blocking the way. There will be a prominent band that is part of the trouble; cut it with a blade or scissors until you feel it release. If there is a coronary artery in that territory, don't for heaven's sake cut it. Releasing the outflow tract will make it easier to see whole margin of the VSD. Closing it is the next job.

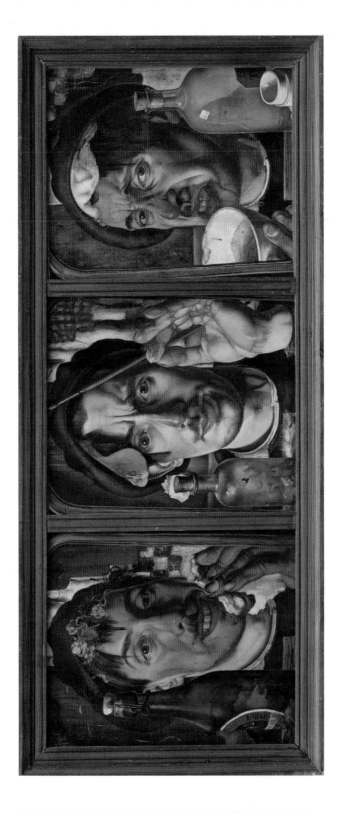

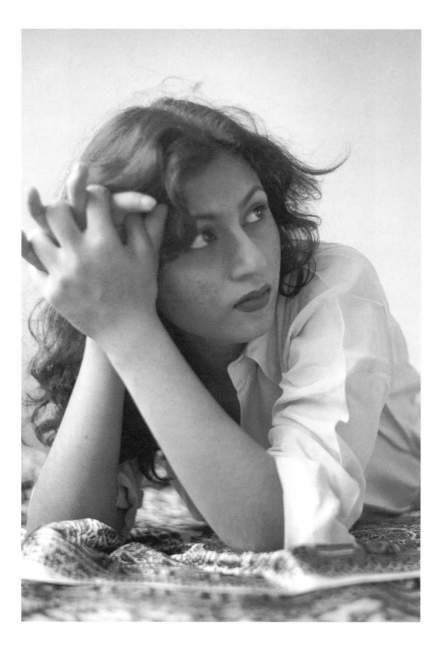

Previous page: Confined by desperate fatigue, the artist Dick Ket painted self-portraits. Looking in his mirror with forensic honesty, he documented his physical deterioration due to chronic lack of oxygen, likely caused by tetralogy of Fallot. (Note his 'clubbed' fingertips, a common feature among 'blue' children.) Ket started his series of portraits in the 1920s; these ones were unfinished when he died in 1940.

Above: The Indian actress Madhubala in 1951, aged eighteen. *Life* magazine's glamour-shoot shows her star quality; the picture was taken just before her first health crisis due to her Eisenmenger's syndrome. Even seventeen years before her death, Madhubala's clubbed fingernails are just distinguishable and her lipstick is working to disguise her blueness.

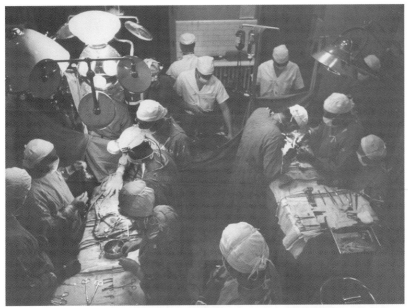

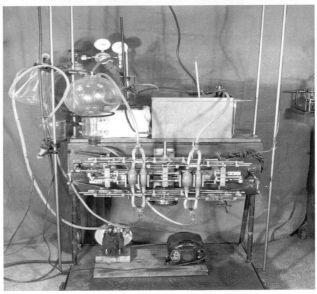

Top: A cross-circulation operation viewed from the dome, University of Minnesota, 1954; this is the hospital where Mickey Shaw's groundbreaking operation was performed the same year. On the operating table to the left, surgeons surround a child (Marsha Gilliam) whose Ventricular Septal Defect they are to close; Dr Lillehei is wearing a headlight. On the right is Marsha's mother, Mary, being prepared to support her daughter's circulation.

Above: A heart-lung machine used in Toronto, Canada, between 1951 and 1956. Such machines were developed to keep the patient alive during open-heart surgery. Visible are four monkey lungs which the child's blood would be pumped through to keep it oxygenated. Of twenty-eight children operated on this way, only three survived – though not all the problems related to the shortcomings of the heart-lung machine.

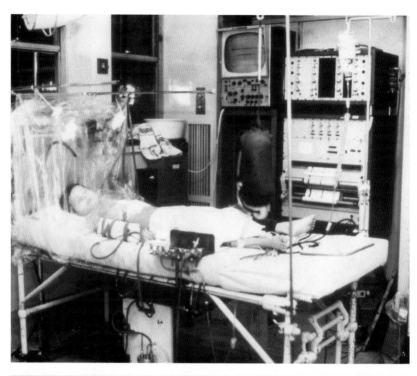

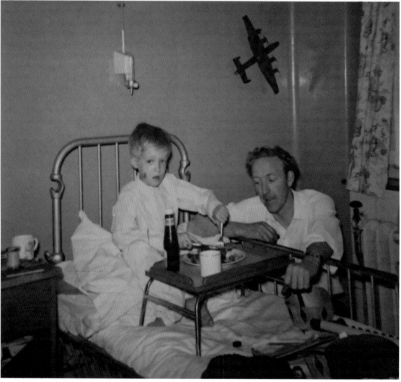

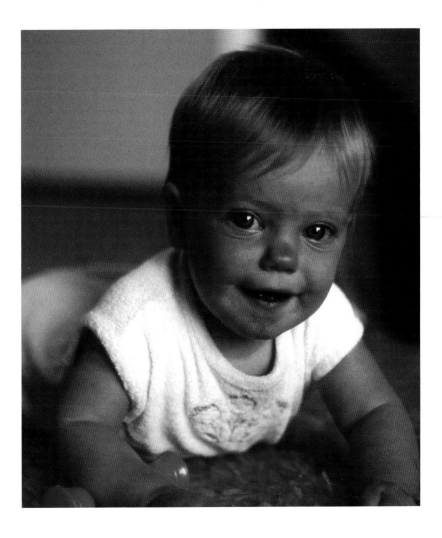

Opposite, top: A child recovering from an operation at Great Ormond Street Hospital in the mid 1970s. The child is breathing for himself with his head inside an oxygen tent. The development of intensive care units in the mid twentieth century was crucial for improving survival rates of children who had undergone surgery.

Opposite, bottom: Barry Butler with his father Ron, in the Hammersmith Hospital, London, 1962. Barry was in hospital for six months on a men's ward; he saw few other children in the hospital during that time. For a while he had a tracheostomy so he could not talk. Every evening he wrote down his breakfast order: Rice Krispies, banana, half a slice of toast and half a slice of bread.

Above: Tiffiney Schmohe, a 'blue baby'. Born in 1971 with Transposition of the Great Vessels, Tiffiney was the first survivor of a 'Mustard' operation at Colorado General Hospital, Denver. Later she graduated from university, travelled and worked abroad, and is now the mother of two boys. She is a member of the 'Mustard and Senning Survivors Facebook Group'. Social media offers a powerful modern tool for patients to exchange essential – sometimes lifesaving – information.

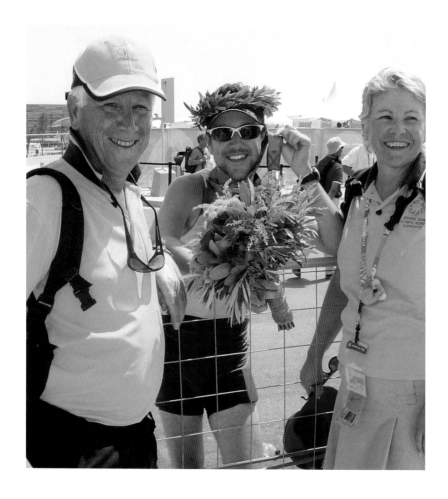

Above: Michael Toon was born in Brisbane, Australia, with Transposition of the Great Arteries. He had a 'Senning' operation in 1983 and has been 'happily healthy since (have had a few pacemakers, but who hasn't!)'. Michael qualified in medicine but here, with his parents, he shows off the bronze medal he won in the 2004 Athens Olympics, where he was coxswain for the Australian Men's Heavyweight Rowing Eight.

Opposite: Three siblings. Q. Can you tell which has had an arduous series of three open-heart operations for their single ventricle condition? A. Tia, the youngest. Thanks also to Josh and Caitlin.

Following page: A portrait of Liza Morton from the 'Scarred for Life' exhibition, 2015. Liza has been reliant on pacemakers since birth. Her body and limbs show countless scars, each corresponding to a setback – broken wires, new batteries. In this photograph we see one scar from open-heart surgery (age twelve) and another under her collarbone, where her body has hosted several pacemakers. Liza is now a psychologist and a mother.

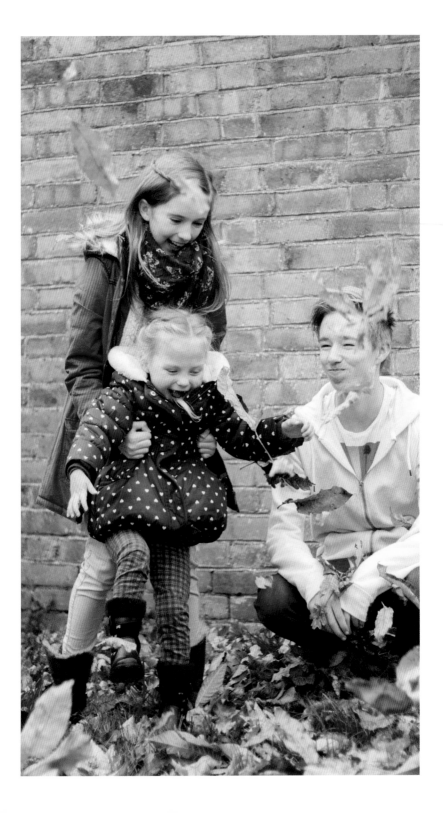

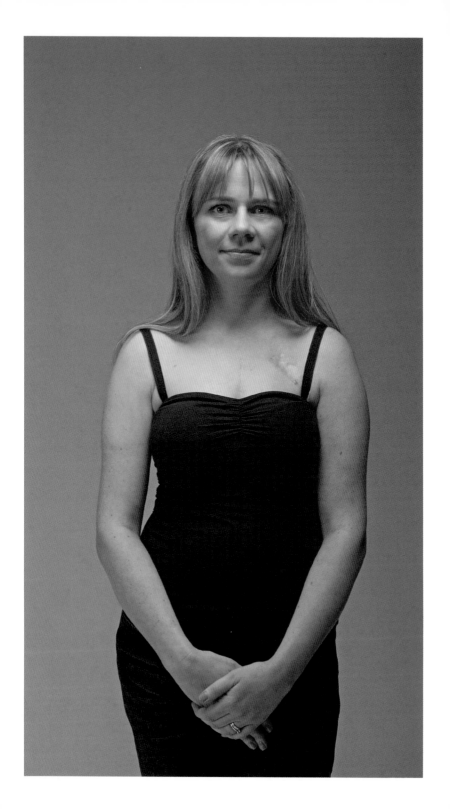

Take a double-armed, pledgetted suture.* The thread will be made of a smooth monofilament synthetic polymer and it will be already crimped into an eyeless needle by the manufacturer; needle and thread are in-line so that their passage through delicate tissue is atraumatic.† You cannot hope to use your own hands to work down this deep hole. Use one of those nifty needle holders that you grip in your fingertips like forceps; no need now for those clumsy ones held in your palm and operated like scissors. The needles are less than 1cm long and curved, so that the small movement of rotating your wrist will complete the stitch. With standard forceps in your left hand, start stitching at 12 o'clock from where you are standing, away from the margin of the hole; bring both stitches out towards you and settle the pledgets on the ventricular septum. Cut a patch to the right size – Goretex or bovine pericardium, your choice. Put both needles through the patch, lower the patch into the defect and tie it down. This is an important knot. Next, stitch around the defect starting in the area of the aortic valve, which you must avoid, and working towards you. Stitch by stitch through the septum and the patch until you reach the tricuspid valve. Bring your stitch through the tricuspid valve close to its supporting ring and put a clip on that end of the suture while you return to the other needle. Now using the other needle go stitch by stitch around the defect to the right; this time it is the conducting system you need to avoid; anchor your patch away from the area between

---

* One thread, curved needles at each end, with two little 'felt' squares already sewn through the thread; the 'pledgets' help avoid the sutures tearing through tissue.

† Gone are the days of needles with eyes being threaded by the scrub nurse – though this is how Lillehei's nurse mounted the needles for Mickey Shaw's Fallot repair. The bulkiest part of a needle you thread at home is at the eye where there are also two thicknesses of thread. In use, this leaves a hole that is not completely filled by the single thread you leave when you pull the needle through. Atraumatic needles are eyeless.

tricuspid valve and muscle. This section is tricky as you may need to weave in and out of the strings that support the tricuspid valve. Also if you or your assistant pull too hard on the suture, things tear; you will probably need to support the suture line, perhaps with a strip of pericardium to avoid 'cheese-wiring' through the valve. Now you are back to the place you left the other end of the suture. Tie them both down together through the reinforcing strip. The VSD is closed.

Next you need to attend again to the outflow tract; there will still be some obstruction to deal with, at the pulmonary valve or above it or below it – or all three. It's usually best to open the pulmonary artery to get a good look at the valve from above. A bit of 'plastic surgery' here is probably in order – if the valve leaflets are fused together, split them apart; if the base of the leaflets are stuck to the wall of the artery, release them. Get help from your assistant to look up into the outflow tract from below; they will have to retract the tricuspid valve again to help you do this. You need to assess if carving out muscle in the area under the valve will be enough to relieve the blockage or whether you are going to need to enlarge the area with a patch. By pushing a calibrated probe through your opened-up outflow tract, check if your resection is sufficient – tables document how big is 'big enough' for a child of any particular size. Assuming you have done enough, the end is in sight and the perfusionists can start to rewarm blood and body.

Soon you will be ready to let the heart fill up again, which will make it want to beat. But before you let it take over actually pumping blood out to the body, you need to be certain there is absolutely no air left inside the heart – bubbles in the blood can block vessels in the brain or the coronaries just as surely as clots can. While they are rewarming, close any hole between the atria (many Fallots have one) and de-air the left side of the heart by letting it fill up with blood. With the left and right hearts separated, you can take the clamp off the aorta so that warm blood is running down the coronary arteries, provoking the heart to beat again. The right heart also gradually fills, blood displacing the air. The anaesthetist can start ventilating the lungs.

Now the perfusionsist can divert less blood away from the heart, letting it fill enough to eject blood out. The anaesthetist's monitors will tell if there is enough blood flow through the lungs and the arterial blood pressure trace can be monitored; if everyone is happy that the heart is coping, you come off bypass. This is likely to be completely straightforward, no stone heart, no alarming rhythm problems. Around now, it will be worth looking at your repair with the echo probe that the anaesthetist situated in the gullet, behind the heart; a cardiologist can come in and check that there is no residual hole between the ventricles and that the outflow tract looks respectable. When all has been well for a few minutes you can set about taking out the tubes connecting the body to the machinery that has been doing its work, starting with one of the venous lines and ending with the aortic cannula. Tie down all the purse strings.

Begin to close the chest. Drag two plastic drain tubes inwards through skin incisions, position them below and in front of the heart and put heavy stitches in the skin to hold them in place; if there is going to be bleeding after the chest is closed, at least it will come out through these tubes. Take the retractor out. Close the sternum with strong braided sutures (or with wires if you must). Using absorbable sutures, cover the bone with the layer of tissue immediately below the skin. Finally close the skin carefully with winding back-and-forth buried sutures leaving a clean line of skin apposed to skin. Check everyone is happy and let the team move the patient to the ward.

Helpful hints: choose an experienced scrub nurse, someone who will give you the instrument you need, not necessarily the one you ask for. Tell people what you are doing next, not what you are doing now. Focus – keep your eye on the job, other people can follow the monitors. If something goes wrong, all your training suddenly becomes important to the solution of the problem. You can't solve it an hour later, or tomorrow. Nor can you go to the library and look it up.

★   ★   ★

If you want to get a surgeon to talk, ask them about how they learned to tie a knot; it's an entry-level skill, a craft not learned in lectures. Each will tell you how they procured several yards of suture material and spent the night tying knots to armchairs, tables, dogs, cats, fellow students and anything else that was handy. The particular surgeon explaining here learned knots when he was an English medical student visiting a Southern US state – ostensibly to learn surgery but mainly sampling the novel party scene. It was a time of social unrest locally and the Emergency Room was busy – to the extent that another pair of hands could be quite useful. His mentor told him to learn knots and this was his apprenticeship regime.

Tying surgical knots (you might like to try this at home):

> Learn the single-handed knot, left-handed and single-handed knot, right-handed.
> Learn the double-handed knot, left-handed and double-handed knot, right-handed. (There are dozens of websites that will take you through the sequence.)

> Put on surgical gloves that are one size too small and on top of those a pair that are one size too big (you will lose much of the feedback from your fingertips, leaving you on 'automatic pilot'). Repeat the above, single left, single right, double left, double right.

> Repeat the above with Vaseline on your gloves.

Repeat the above with a blindfold on.

Repeat the above with your hands behind your back.

Repeat the above with your hands under water.

Repeat the above with slippery suture materials.

You may now enter the emergency room where the next step is to understand that tying knots onto living tissue is not like tying knots around the arms of chairs.

Surgeons work down deep holes, often unable to see what they are doing because blood is filling the chest or abdomen or skull, where invisible slippery organs lurk and where it is imperative that the knots do not come undone.

If you enjoy all this, perhaps you have the makings of a surgeon.

11

This won't hurt a bit: recovery

According to his father, Guy had been a serious and rather charming child – very blue all his young life. Over the years, Guy had made many visits to hospital; they had often been difficult and rather frightening. He had come to realize that the arrival of a small toy when his dad came home from work was an advance warning of another hospital visit. In 1982, when he was nine, the coveted Star Wars Millennium Falcon Lego kit arrived in a big box; Guy was elated. Tearful himself, his father asked, 'Do you know why you are getting this?' In fact, Guy had known instantly – both that he was to go to hospital and that this admission was to be the 'big one'.

His parents had always talked straightforwardly to him. He knew that he needed an operation to grow up and was bright enough to understand that otherwise he wouldn't. Since he was about seven, they had all found a way to talk about death – and about bravery (decades later, Guy was ready with his father's quote from Julius Caesar: 'Cowards die many times before their deaths. The valiant never taste of death but once'). They travelled as a team on the long journey to London – in it together. Heading into the operation, Guy could see that his parents were terribly sad and he felt it his duty to do his bit to cheer them up. 'See you in a minute,' he said as he disappeared out of view.

His mother and father spent the day in a churchyard and 'thought about stuff'. Telling me all this thirty-five years later, his father silently fought to keep his composure as he described the 'thrilling' moment when, after taking in the tableau of his son – barely recognizable with tubes and trappings all over his face – he noticed that the toes peeping out of the sheets were pink.

I have been reminded many times that nothing prepares you for your first sight of your own child laid out on a bed in the intensive care unit (ICU) – 'the worst thing I've ever had to see in my life,' said one mother. The relief that they are alive at all is brilliant, but there is something about the scene that brings home the fact that an ICU is not a place of safety. It isn't – and never more so than now. In the 'old days,' deaths used to happen on the operating table and now this is extremely rare. These days, deaths happen in the ICU to children who you may have glanced at as you walked past, to families you may have nodded to in the corridor.

*   *   *

At the beginning of cardiac surgery for children, there was no concept of 'intensive care'. After surgery, a child would be propped up in bed with a drip in their arm and a pipe coming out of their chest. If they were asleep, you might have to look carefully at their breathing to even know if they were alive – there were no monitors to glance up at. A nurse and a junior doctor might have been delegated to look after them – though apart from transfusing blood to replace what was coming out of the drainage tube, there was little they could do. Parents were nowhere to be seen. Gradually the surroundings changed, an expert workforce was established, the technology completely transformed – and now parents are doing long shifts at the bedside.

The concept of 'intensive care' as a 'place to recuperate in' originated in the polio epidemics of the late 1940s and early 1950s. Polio paralyses and, if the muscles of the chest are hit, doctors need to take over patients' breathing for days at a time if the victim is to have any chance of recovering. The need for a ward where lots of dependent patients could be supported together, for twenty-four-hour vigilance, for teamwork, for nurses willing to deal with complexity and drama – as well as practical experience of taking over the breathing of a human body for days at a time – all these were first figured out during those epidemics.

In the US epidemic of 1952, some of Minnesota's polio patients were cared for just one floor below the State's first children having open-heart operations. Those patients were few and when the operation was over, there was no special place to send them – they would simply return to the beds they had left earlier. For the first twenty-four hours an experienced nurse might be hired from an agency and there might be some doctors fretting nearby. As heart operations became more established, and to shield the other children on the ward from the sights and sounds of tension and distress, the next step was to kit out surgical recovery rooms* to accommodate patients for their first post-operative night; the precedent that post-operative cardiac patients needed one-to-one nursing day and night was set at around this time. Then, as the numbers of cardiac surgery patients escalated further, intensive care wards as we now recognize them began to be built.

Through the 1960s, children and adults would often be accommodated on the same post-operative ward. This was a little exciting for one boy who, at fourteen years of age, got his first glimpse of a female breast, but most people remember the open-plan and rather 'veterinary' atmosphere of those times as very distressing.

---

* The French name 'salles de réanimation' evokes the atmosphere of a recovery room.

As surgeons began to specialize, congenital heart operations came to be consolidated in fewer centres where competence could be fostered and the next generation of surgeons trained. For example, Mary Jane's family was advised to drive her all the way from New Hampshire to Birmingham, Alabama for her major repair. In 1973, the Alabama service was internationally respected and very busy. Its intensive care facility was like a huge factory floor, stark and cold, with twelve beds on each side of the room. Mary Jane was almost thirteen years old, starting to develop breasts and pubic hair. 'The nurses and doctors made me lay in the bed with no clothes on, most of the time without even a sheet covering me. I was very embarrassed and for the first twenty-four hours after surgery I couldn't even talk since I was still intubated. My parents could only visit twice a day for fifteen minutes.'*

Fast-forward to the present time and the physical layout of current ICUs. These strive – with various degrees of success – to serve as a child's bedroom (cuddly toys propping up crucial pipes), an office (the nurse's computer workspace), a showcase for modern medical technology (the sometimes incredible banks of equipment at a small baby's bedside) and a place for a parent to relax (the chair is provided, but we all know that there is more to relaxation than comfort). No picture of the built environment conveys its unique soundscape (beeps, chirps, alarms and the to-and-fro noise of assisted breathing) or smellscape (the tang of cleanliness and antiseptic lotion) – or the palpable emotional atmosphere. It is as if the area around each bed is a micro-climate: here the sun is shining (over a bed where a child is forging ahead), there it's flat calm (in a side-room where machines are doing a lot of work for a very

---

* 'I have always been a visual person, which can sometimes work to my disadvantage. I remember every detail of every hospitalization. Many years of psychological therapy have helped me to be able to discuss these memories without re-traumatizing myself.'

sick baby who is perhaps imperceptibly improving), over there fog
is rolling in (for a family receiving awful news) – and around the
nurses' station there may be banter as in any other workplace. Every
now and then a 'weather front' engulfs the whole ICU: people in
scrubs hurry in, visitors hustle out and surgeons with full lights
and sterility operate on a patient in the open ward – and everyone
knows that someone's child is in mortal danger. ICU is not for the
faint-hearted – not for staff, not parents, not patients.

★ ★ ★

Even an operation that has transformed a heart's performance successfully can often leave the whole body reeling from the trauma
of the surgery, so the early recovery period can be very unstable.
During the late 1940s, the know-how for undertaking 'outside
the heart' operations was being shared (shunts, repairing narrow
aortas) and the 1950s recorded 'firsts' for the open-heart repairs
of many defects. But the phrase 'the operation was a success but
the patient died' was also very current. The first child having a
Ventricular Septal Defect (VSD) repair died a few days after the
operation, which took place in Minnesota in 1954 when the child
was thirteen months old. So did the first having a baffle operation
for Transposition of the Great Arteries (see page 277), which took
place in New Orleans in 1956 when the child was nine months
old. Their autopsies showed that their operations had 'worked',
but these two skinny little babies with massive chest incisions
(armpit-to-armpit) and no ventilator to support them simply could
not cope with breathing for themselves. Their nurses and surgeons
had to watch them slowly die in their beds. To grasp how primitive
the care of small babies was in those early days, bear in mind that
even in 1963, Patrick Bouvier Kennedy, the US president's own
son, was born early weighing 2.1kg and died two days later of
his prematurity. Babies born at this weight do need some expert
care, but then it simply did not exist; for the past three decades,

virtually all babies born so small have survived and can now even have successful heart surgery.*

The learning curve linking then and now has comprised many, many small steps that have contributed vastly to the (relative) safety of heart surgery for contemporary children. Along with the notion of ICUs has come a huge range of drugs and technology and specialist staff whose business it is to know how to use them.

The origins of intensive care as a 'body of medical knowledge' are also found in the mid-century polio epidemics. In the 1953 Copenhagen polio epidemic, there were days when seventy patients in a single hospital needed support for their breathing. For some polio victims, a leg first becomes floppy then, sometimes over hours, the paralysis can move up their bodies, knocking out the muscles of the chest wall. If you hold your chest absolutely still, you become aware of breathing only with your diaphragm. You cannot cough effectively. Lose diaphragmatic movement too and you watch yourself suffocate and die. But the paralysis of polio can recover, provided the patient can be tided over while their immune system finds and disables the virus that lurks in their spinal cord. During the outbreaks, the machine of choice for taking over a patient's breathing for days or weeks was the 'iron lung'.† The problem was that polio is an extremely infectious virus and in an epidemic there were not always enough iron lungs to go around. The doctors needed another plan.

The Copenhagen regime was to do a tracheostomy (make

* 2.1kg is just under 5 pounds. 'Low birth-weight' is defined at 2.5kg, about 5½ pounds. By 2011, a Californian group were reporting that nine out of ten babies who had the double jeopardy of low birth-weight and cardiac surgery were alive one year later.
† The patient's body is laid in a metal and glass 'pod' with his head sticking out as from a sleeping bag. A vacuum pump rhythmically sucks air out of the chamber. If the patient's neck is properly sealed, this 'negative pressure ventilation' makes his chest expand and he 'breathes in'. The actress Mia Farrow spent time in an iron lung at the age of nine; she said it was 'the end of my childhood'.

a hole in the patient's neck, just below their larynx),* position a short curved tube pointing down the airway towards the lungs (tracheostomy tube), hook the tube up to a squeeze-bag and pay a medical student £1.50 per shift to squeeze the bag. This could go on for weeks. If the medical student did not squeeze enough, the patient would drift off to 'sleep' as the waste-gas called carbon dioxide accumulated in their blood; squeeze too much and the patient would develop pins and needles, anxiety and jittery vision.† The wards where these unfortunate patients were cared for served as laboratories for learning about long-term ventilation.

For the first decade of children's heart surgery, the anaesthetist would put a breathing tube through the child's mouth into their windpipe and take over their breathing during the operation by squeezing a bag in the circuit – then simply take the tube out at the end. There was no 'breathing machine' and no army of medical students to squeeze the bags (iron lungs would have sucked the recently sewn-up chest apart.) The child would simply have to manage to breathe and cough on their own, despite the post-anaesthetic sedation, despite the pain in their chests and despite the secretions in their lungs. For many frail, exhausted children, this was simply too much to expect.

Having learned the hard way, when later surgeons anticipated that a child might have difficulty coughing, they would put in a tracheostomy tube before leaving the operating room. The work of

---

* The larynx is the Adam's apple. The trachea extends between the back of the throat down to the chest where it divides into two bronchi, one for each lung. The larynx is the area in the neck supporting the vocal cords where the voice is generated. Air has to pass upwards through the cords to make a sound.
† These symptoms correspond to deviations from normal in the acid/alkali levels in the blood. Copenhagen was a good place to learn about 'acid/base' (pH) balance in blood because even in 1953, the Carlsberg manufacturers were already tracking pH levels in their lager and adapted their equipment to monitor patients' blood levels.

breathing through your neck is a little less than breathing through your nose, simply because the pathway is shorter, but this was not the main reason for the additional operation. A hole in a child's neck gives nurses the route to suck out any lung secretions that the child does not have the energy to cough up herself. Children resist this suctioning with all their strength; they have to be held down. But a tracheostomy tube also stops air from heading up past the vocal cords, so the child's distress and protest is completely silent.

Without a 'breathing machine,' oxygen was the only other panacea that could realistically be offered to 'support' a patient, and if you had visited an early ICU you would have seen people in oxygen tents. Children would wake up shrouded in a clear plastic canopy which covered the whole bed and was accessed from outside though a zip – from inside there was no escape. Oxygen from cylinders beside the bed would be piped through crushed ice to cool and humidify the space inside.

When I first arrived in the heart wards of a children's hospital in the late 1970s, oxygen tents were just on their way out. At the time, I had thought of the tent as a child's place of safety, perhaps because patients became so apprehensive when I opened the zip. As with so many assumptions, I never checked it out with the children themselves. Many patients I have spoken to – Alan, Judith, Laura, Steve, Nick, indeed everyone who remembered their oxygen tent – had found it alien and utterly ghastly. They had spent endless hours in its damp, oppressive and extremely lonely interior. Susan was nine and on her ward in 1961 London there was a complete embargo on family visiting, but the ward staff had grown fond of her during her many admissions. So when she first came round after her operation, disorientated, frightened, claustrophobic and damp, a big black hand slipped inside the tent and held hers. The ward cleaning lady had sat up into the night so as to be there when Susan woke up.

Judith's operation was in 1968 and she still remembers her rising panic when she came to in her tent with both arms splinted straight. That horror was nothing compared to the realization that she could not speak. Inexplicably, she could move her lips but no sound came out. What had happened to her voice? Nobody had explained about having a tracheostomy – and she could not ask. It crossed her eight-year-old mind that this was forever.

These days, children and adults are usually sedated for at least the first few post-operative hours while their circulation settles and a ventilator does the breathing for them. Over the past thirty years, ventilators have become very sophisticated, with sensors that synchronize with any breathing effort the patient is making and fail-safe gizmos that avoid dangerous swings of pressure. These ventilators push air and oxygen rhythmically into the lungs. The earliest machines developed during the mid 1950s were ad hoc inventions, using bellows and windscreen-wiper motors, but commercial corporations soon took up the necessary 'research and development'. The most successful US ventilator for a couple of decades was the Bird Mark 7 Respirator, known to its friends as 'the Bird' – mother of 'baby Bird' which became widely available in 1970 for ventilating babies and which might have saved the President's son.

In fact, had you visited an early ICU, you would rarely have seen a baby. Until well into the 1960s, it was mainly middle-sized children who had open-heart surgery; a surgeon's customary courage often failed when faced with a smaller child. This was partly the physical challenge of their size (remember a child's heart is only as big as his own fist); babies' blood vessels are also tiny, which is challenging for the anaesthetist. Taking over their respiration with a breathing bag or an early ventilator was also dicey – too much pressure could easily burst a lung. Perhaps because they were so evidently fragile, it was simply more acceptable for a specialist to quietly tell parents that their baby needed to reach a certain age or weight before an operation could be contemplated – knowing that, for many diagnoses, only a tiny minority would survive that long.

Nowadays if you visit a cardiac ICU, more than half the patients you see will be infants, many less than one month old. As they arrive back from their operations – and even if things are going well – you are likely to find these babies on a big bed, still and unresponsive in the middle of an enormous web of stickers, wires, tubes and tapes. There will be a fat tube pushed down one nostril and pointing into their lungs (connecting the child to a ventilator) and another tube in the other nostril going down to drain their stomach. There will probably be two slimmer tubes in their neck (through which fluids and drugs are slowly pumped into the circulation) and another in a wrist or leg artery (monitoring the blood pressure and generating the see-saw wiggly lines you see on a cardiac monitor). There will be a thermometer sensor passed through their mouth or nose (measuring 'core temperature') and another stuck to a hand or foot (measuring 'peripheral temperature'). A tube goes into the bladder (monitoring urine flow) and at least two more come out of their chest to drain out any blood that has been gradually seeping out from stitch holes inside. There will be at least two wires coming out through their skin (to be hooked up to a pacemaker if heart rhythms become a problem). As well as these twelve-plus wires and tubes coming out of their bodies, there will be ECG stickers (monitoring the heart rhythm) and an oxygen monitor on a finger or toe. If the baby has already caused concern in the operating room, they may have a tube in their abdomen ready to dialyse for transient kidney failure. If a baby has already been precarious, the surgeon may be concerned that its swollen heart would be too cramped if its chest were closed. This means that a few parents return to see their babies lying on the bed with a big notice reading 'open chest', warning everyone that, underneath the bandages, the baby's breastbone is still gaping open and the beating of the heart may be weirdly visible through the dressings.

Some of these tubes are 'doing stuff' – the ventilator 'does' the breathing and the 'intravenous lines' deliver the drugs; but most are there for monitoring. Changes – fast or slow – chart the patient's recovery, or may anticipate a crisis. Much of the expertise of ICU physicians entails reading the drift of many, many numbers. If the trend is good, they will pace the dismantling of all the ICU paraphernalia perfectly – all of those twenty-plus tubes and wires will come out in ones or twos until the child can be lifted off the bed for her first tentative cuddle. If the drift of the numbers is tricky, there are usually several options to try to avert a crisis – the proverbial 'two steps back' – more drugs, more equipment, more tests.

ICU doctors always prefer to avert a crisis but occasionally, as in TV soaps, drama comes out of the blue. Usually the patient is unconscious when emergencies happen, but Christina was almost ready to leave the ward when suddenly she felt an overwhelming pain – 'too much to cope with' – and had difficulty breathing. In moments she was aware of nurses and doctors surrounding her bed. In rapid succession, she was very scared then very drowsy. The nurse by her head was saying 'Christina, stay with us'. She opened her eyes once on the way to the operating theatre; it was like a purple moving tunnel. Waking up later in the ICU again, her immediate thought was 'I'm back'. She had experienced a pneumothorax; outside air had got into her chest cavity, perhaps through a chest-drain hole, and its volume had expanded with every breath, compressing her lung and probably cramming her heart into a smaller and smaller space.

★   ★   ★

For parents, the time in intensive care is a time of great anxiety. From the very first days of her daughter Sarah's life, Connie had made it her mission to keep her baby alive until she could have her big operation. The next eighteen months were pervaded by horrible anxiety; Connie was ever vigilant. The operation when it came was very long. Connie takes over the story:

We were in the ICU waiting room during shift change, and heard our surgeon and cardiologist called over the loud-speaker 'to 4400 stat' [Latin: *statim*, immediately]. We knew that was the ICU, and we knew our daughter was the only heart baby there at the time. We ran down the hall, and saw them slide the board under her and hold the paddles over her. Then they saw us at the doorway, and we were taken to a room just outside the unit. But in that moment, I fully understood that all my actions and attempts to protect her had not amounted to anything. It was an epiphany. She never belonged to me. Those eighteen months might be all I ever had, and I had spent too many of them in fear and anger at God. Seems like a sort of fiction, I know, but it really was that clear and evident to me. I promised myself and God that I would never make that mistake again.

Her daughter survived. We meet her again in the last chapter.

These days, hospitals make great efforts to accommodate par-ents in the vicinity of their children and this has been a civilizing influence for all sides. Children behave better – and doctors behave better – when parents are around. But there once was a time when parents were not even contactable – even when you really needed them. In 1968, Alan's mother had to stay two difficult bus journeys away from the hospital. Aunty Mags had no telephone, so when her son's wound fell apart on the ward, a policeman had to be dispatched to knock on her door in the evening to tell her to go to the hospital immediately; she barely managed to keep her terror under control after that. (But the boy was stitched up again and remembers being wheeled out onto a balcony to see fireworks for the first time – children's hospitals do make great efforts to leave their patients with some happy memories.)

Geoffrey was a teenager from 'the provinces'; in 1962 he was accommodated on an adult ward and savoured the novelty. The

Middlesex was the nearest teaching hospital to the private-medicine enclave of Harley Street and there was a lot of swishing of chauffeur-driven cars in and out of the car-park. A commissionaire in top hat and tails controlled the reception area. His surgeon was Thomas Holmes Sellors.* The wards were long, serried ranks of beds on each side. Patients, doctors and nurses all smoked on the ward (including sixteen-year-old Geoffrey). After the operation, he had wheelchair races with his pal in the next bed along the extensive corridors, and remembers looking out of the window and seeing Winston Churchill taking the air in the courtyard garden as he recovered from breaking his leg in Monte Carlo.

★ ★ ★

In a busy modern children's cardiac ICU, roughly half the patients will have moved on to a lower-dependency ward by about the fourth day after their operation. Undoubtedly these first days are stressful for their families, but at least they have had an encouraging forward momentum. Some children are technology-dependent for much longer, however, and for their parents the ICU days can assume a different quality. Babies with Hypoplastic Left Heart Syndrome (HLHS) are born with only a right ventricle to depend on for their survival. An urgent and high-risk operation has to be

---

* Holmes Sellors' surgical mentor, Sir Gordon Gordon-Taylor, offered a view of the Middlesex surgeon's life: 'The surgeon's day is a twenty-four-hour day, and necessarily I have developed some curious formulae in my creed: I have never tested the allure of the cinema, although on occasion I do enjoy a theatre; I have never had the time nor the slightest desire to play bridge; I have never been a Freemason or driven a car with my own hands; I have never done a crossword puzzle, been in a pub or drunk a drop of beer or, since infancy, milk; I do not smoke. I have hardly ever attended a committee or council, save those connected with the Royal College of Surgeons of England, which are regarded by all as sacrosanct, and I have never taken a holiday that lasted more than two days. Therefore, my life has at least been a most happy and perhaps a useful one.'

attempted in the first days of life if there is to be any future – this is 'stage 1' of three operations a child with HLHS will need in early childhood to achieve a stable circulation. Because of prenatal ultrasound screening, over half the parents of children with HLHS have had forewarning of the need for surgery and naturally are tremendously relieved to see their babies back in ICU after the operation. But they are perhaps less prepared for the next part of the ordeal. The death rate for the 'stage 1' operation has gone down over the years, at least partly due to improved ICU care. But the flip side of that statement is that few survivors of 'stage 1' HLH surgery go through intensive care without some setback. In a big US review of almost two thousand newborns having 'stage 1' surgery, half were in hospital for more than twenty-five days and some for considerably longer. Surrounded by kindly staff, their parents endure a subtle and very modern form of torture, never off-duty, maintaining their vigil.

This is how one mother speaks for those parents:

> Looking back, all my memories blur into a wash of sitting by his bedside, day after day, with him looking utterly still and spread out, so unlike a baby – more like a frog on a dissecting table – puffy with fluid, wan, completely immobile, and with all the gentle beepings and bongings of a myriad machines constantly going on in the background. The staff in ICU are wonderful, words can't express how good – not just unremitting in their care, but *cheerful*, positive, and even endowed with a sense of humour – something I really came to appreciate.

It's best that these parents get on well with the staff, as they will be back by their child's bedside at least twice more, for 'stages 2 and 3'.

Another recurring story that parents tell of their time in hospital is how complete strangers are so ready to offer help when they hear of their predicament. Gill and her family were 200 miles from home with baby Michael having 'stage 1' surgery. A parking attendant noticed them daily in the rather expensive car-park near the hospital. As soon as he learned about their son, he made it his business to save a parking spot in that permanently full place, free of charge, for all the weeks they were there. They were put up in accommodation established by a charitable trust set up by parents of a child who had died of cancer. Its fridge was supplied daily by a supermarket chain that is a household name in England and volunteers would bake a cake at 4 p.m. every day. Granny was looked after by contacts of the Church of England Mothers' Union. A prayer chain letter had the whole family – and their surgeon – prayed for by 'Episcopalians, Presbyterians – including the current and several past moderators of the Church of Scotland – Wee Frees, Methodists, Catholics – including Pluscarden Abbey – and also by communities of Jews, Muslims, Hindus, Ba'hais and Buddhists. We found, within only a few weeks, we were being prayed for in places and by people we'd scarcely heard of, let alone encountered.' People care.

★   ★   ★

Lately I have spent time with many 'graduates' of cardiac intensive care. There was curiosity on both sides. I could answer many questions that they had never been able to ask, and they could paint a very different picture of a scene I thought I knew well. We all know how tricky memory can be: how we forget what we did yesterday, yet remember with exquisite clarity an inconsequential moment in childhood. We know that what we remember may not be exactly what we witnessed, and how memory can make out a thing to have been much more than it was. At the time, these people may have been tired and emotional. There may have been some mind-altering drugs in their systems. Yet as I listened to patients' vivid memories of their decades-past ICU stays, I have surely to accept that what these people have so candidly offered really has been their mental diary of that part of their lives.

Everyone mentions the pain – I know one surgeon who warns his adult patients that cardiac surgery is like being in a car-crash without a seatbelt. Here is one man's description of waking up from an adult operation:

> With absolutely no sense of the passing of time, light opens up and you are in another place. There are voices. Quickly relief, and also pain, a sense of self, a need to hang on. You feel groggy, as though you have been in the sun too long. Actually you are in a bed but because all your sensations are muddled, it feels like a cocoon. Pain anchors you. You feel some sort of responsibility to be alive. Sounds are more important than vision. Beeps. There is a sense that this is real – but you also imagine things, though you sort of know they aren't true. [Bedouin tribesmen happened to be sitting on the floor at the end of his bed . . .]

Those who had operations as adults had all gone down to the operating room knowing that if they were to wake up at all, it would be in an ICU bed with a nurse nearby. Not so for the children; many youngsters had no idea where they were when they first surfaced. Several had thought that the operation was somehow still happening. Children's heart surgery had been well established for almost twenty years before anyone thought seriously about preparing children for the experience they would return to. In no era does a young child wake up, pinioned to a bed with inexplicable tubes coming out of their bodies, and think 'This is for my own good.' They feel violated.

Bernhard, then aged seven, remembers surfacing in a strange cot, feeling utterly abandoned and gazing down at his body. He was tied down by tubes in both ankles, both elbows, another in his tummy – and some sort of wire. Nobody had explained to Bernhard any more than they would to a dog. In his sixties now, he remembers being silently stunned. There is something appalling about seeing a tube coming out of your chest and dripping red stuff into a jar on the floor – even adults sometimes feel faint at the sight of blood. The rational explanation for these drains, stuck into every chest after every operation, is that continuing bleeding is better out than in – but the visceral revulsion of seeing bloody pipes coming out of a child's body does not come from a rational place.

Perhaps because of the drugs in their systems, perhaps because of our minds' capacity to bury difficult memories, both children and adults often forget much of their time in ICU beds, even though they appeared lucid to others at the time. But bodies seem to have a capacity for another sort of memory – one that is physically felt and hard ever to put into words. Some people mention experiencing alarming 'echoes' of their time in hospital breaking through in everyday life, and a few have been formally diagnosed with Post Traumatic Stress Disorder. But these felt reverberations, mysteriously triggered, can also be uplifting. Some recognized the feeling they had on waking from a second or third operation – a sense of déjà vu, a sort of 'I'm back, I've made it again' – that can well up apparently out of the blue. It is as if their bodies 'know' they have negotiated the space between life and death before, and are glad to be alive.

★ ★ ★

Almost without exception, I have not looked after the people who have helped with this book. For my own part, I hoped to be someone who might recognize what they were talking about, without a doctor-patient relationship getting in the way. At the very outset of our conversations, almost everyone affirmed how grateful they felt to be alive and – until they were certain I had received that message – they often seemed unwilling to talk candidly about how tough it had been. But for me, one of the immense benefits of these exchanges – so different from anything that patients would have with their own doctor – has been the gems that sometimes come at the very end of a long conversation. Occasionally I had the privilege of patients describing to me what Wordsworth called a 'spot of time',* a deceptively trivial event when their senses were heightened – a moment that has reverberated through their life, a sort of epiphany, a moment when possibilities changed.

Here is Susan's. At seventeen, Susan was so blue that she could not walk and talk at the same time. She had received a shunt at three months of age for pulmonary atresia (an extreme of Fallot's tetralogy in which no blood at all reaches the lungs from the heart). Subsequently, the narrative of her whole life had been that she would die before she was twenty. Her parents and teachers had been resigned to letting her go. At seventeen, she had had enough and – defying her mother – consented on her own for an operation that, in her heart, she believed would kill her. Before the operation she said an unemotional goodbye to her family and left instructions for her burial. But she did not die. The post-operative phase had been long and very hard, but one day she was well enough to be pushed out of the hospital in a wheelchair. It was June. The sun was shining in the clearest possible sky. The noises of the city – the taxis – were hugely immediate. Sun felt warm on her skin and the taste of a lemon sorbet ice cream was extraordinary. In that 'spot of time' she felt utterly alive.

Here is Bernhard's transcendent moment, told in gratitude to everybody who contributed to his survival. Despite the operation

---

* 'There are in our existence spots of time,
    That with distinct pre-eminence retain
    A renovating virtue . . .'
Wordsworth later says these moments can have a lasting quality capable of 'lifting us up when we are fallen'.

that had so horrified him when he was seven, Bernhard had been desperately disabled before his 'big operation' in 1961 when he was thirteen. The operation and its aftermath had been an immense and lonely ordeal, but he had felt surrounded with good will and kind nurses. No longer blue, his head had somehow cleared – memories before that operation are few and foggy. Newly able to get about on his own, he remembers walking under his very own steam, past the twin rows of elderly men in their dormitory-style beds to the end of the ward. From there, through the tall windows, he could look out right over London. With the sunlight streaming over him, he felt as though he had been reborn.

12

Finding a new normal: after surgery

On John's sixth birthday in 1954, Sir Russell Brock opened his chest and, working by feel alone, put some sharp scissors through the muscle of the front of John's heart, into the cavity of his right ventricle, wiggled the tips up across his small, stiff pulmonary valve and out into his pulmonary artery, opened the blades a little and – as he withdrew the instrument – scooped out some of the excessive muscle that was blocking the way out of his right ventricle. John had been very blue and could not walk far; he had Fallot's tetralogy and this operation was Brock's first attempt at improving his lung-blood flow.

John was one of nine children born in a rural cottage a couple of hours' train journey away from London, so during the five months that he was in hospital, he saw little of his family. Now in his late sixties, he is happy to play up how he made friends on the hospital ward, but throughout his time there he was never free of a low-level fear. Stitches, drain tubes, needles and alarming 'surprise' tests puncture the buoyancy of any six-year-old. He approached with ambivalence the Maids Morton Convalescent Home where he spent a couple of weeks after leaving hospital. It was only when he walked into his family's familiar front room and saw his new model farm – waiting for him on the table with the sun shining on it – that he knew that the whole ordeal was finally over.

Getting home after major surgery is a joyful milestone that is usually tinged with apprehension. While in hospital, everyone feels vulnerable and dependent on the competence of others; at home, parents and children have suddenly to rely on their own resources.

In both England and the USA, in the 'ancient history' of congenital heart surgery, patients might be sent away for 'convalescence' to build up their strength and confidence after their long hospital admissions. 'It should be a happy, tranquil time . . . A time of readjustment where books and toys and carefully portioned and routined discipline must find their proper places.'* Frankly, I think John would much rather have gone straight home. But for one four-year-old, her convalescent time was a delight – her first ever experience of the countryside – lovely except for the hay fever. Fifty years later, she has vivid memories of having enough energy to be chased on the lawn by a boy in callipers.

In the 1970s, Chloe was a twenty-something mother of two young children when she had surgery in London to close the hole between the collecting chambers of her heart associated with her Ebstein's anomaly.† Because she had no back-up at home, the hospital social worker organized some respite to give her time to recuperate. A nurse put her on a train at Paddington station and she was met at her destination by an ambulance and taken to a nursing home. When the ambulance door opened, the staff were visibly dismayed. It was a real elderly care home. It smelt of wee, and mute old people sat in a circle in the dayroom. Chloe had kept her emotions together throughout her hospital stay, but there she wept.

---

* From an opinion piece in the *Cincinnati Enquirer* 1932, fundraising for a convalescent facility.
† This forced the blue blood to stream correctly through her (still ramshackle) right heart so that her left heart received only red blood.

These days a young woman in England would not be offered the 'luxury' of help with basic nursing after she left hospital; a quick discharge directly to a patient's home has become what every surgical service aspires to do. In 2014, Amelia was twenty-five and her 'going home' was much more typical of present-day experience. She had not been long in hospital after her operation, but was the least-ill patient on the ward when they needed a bed for an emergency case in the operating theatre – in fact, they needed the bed *now*. Amelia and her family were up for it, though flustered by the timing. It was evening and the discharge lounge was already full of people waiting to be collected, so a nurse wheeled her down to Burger King in the foyer. There she waited in her jogging pants and socks for her father to arrive with some shoes. Customers gave her a wide berth; the gap in her shirt exposed an alarming dressing over the middle of her chest.

Back at her parents' house, everyone was exhausted. The *coup de grâce* for the flagging morale was getting on the obligatory surgical stockings before bed. Amelia's mother had washed them and they had turned pink and shrunk. In hospital, nurses had the knack of nonchalantly rolling them onto their patients' legs; Amelia knew what needed to be done but had no energy to do it. Her father and her boyfriend Sam stood by awkwardly while mother and daughter struggled and bickered until frustrated, defeated tears flowed. They all got to bed at 1 a.m. Homecoming did not seem such a relief.

Being driven to her own place a day later, Amelia was deeply apprehensive. She had watched the quiet expertise of the nurses in hospital and knew she did not have the strength to take care of herself, but also seriously wondered if her loved ones were up to it. But she needn't have worried. After the previous night's débâcle, Sam had looked to YouTube for advice on the getting-on of surgical stockings and links had led him to all sorts of home-nursing tips – videos of how to lift a patient up a bed, how to help someone who had fallen to the ground.

Nevertheless, the next days were tough; Amelia and Sam were both silently terrified. Amelia needed him to be nearby when she went to the toilet or the shower. There were new symptoms – palpitations, visual disturbances and a lump in the scar. What to do? There was a helpline service at the hospital, but Amelia hesitated to bother the nurses. She couldn't sleep through the night. The front of her chest felt as if it had a bad case of sunburn. Just when she really needed a cuddle, Sam could barely touch her.

But things gradually got better. Amelia managed to wash the hospital smells out of her hair. Sam's confidence grew. Her parents came to help with cooking, cleaning and shopping. Sam's mother was reassuring about what was under the bandages. Friends started to arrive. Frightened to hug her, they made do with air-kisses and stroking her arm (though they did want to view her scar). Apprehension about going outside had to be overcome, but she achieved her first slow walk to the supermarket.

After these major milestones are passed, there is often a phase of a recovery when batteries are simply recharging; this makes for long, dull days when morale is sometimes low and flat. Then for many people whose hearts have limited them for years, there comes a moment when they realize that not only are they 'getting better', but that they are 'getting better than ever'. Outside again many days later, Sam suddenly said 'Do you realize how fast you're walking?' The two of them stopped in their tracks, suddenly noticing that they were already ahead of Amelia's preoperative energy levels. From that moment, recovery really took off – an exercise bike, a little holiday, a feeling of glee. The extensive scar down the middle of Amelia's chest settled from scabby to red and gradually faded to a thin silvery line (she had nurtured it as though it was a precious potted plant, cleaning it carefully and rubbing in creams). Sam thought it was sexy. During those long-drawn-out days when there was almost too much time to think, Amelia got to reflecting about how someone had been rummaging around inside her body and that this little scar was all there was to show for it. That this was her secret – that something 'magnificent' had happened. Amelia and Sam began to plan their wedding.

Gentle, bookish Sam, who had started off feeling so hesitant, had become more confident. He had navigated the ordeal for both of them, taking charge in his considerate way. A parent of a fragile infant has to take even greater responsibility when their child eventually gets home. Babies may still have difficulty feeding; there are complicated drug regimes and daily measurements that need charting. We have met Gill before, the mother of Michael who, when he left hospital, was still fed through a tube after his first Hypoplastic Left Heart operation. She tells it how it was:

> For a number of weeks when we were first home, the average feed routine for Michael went something like this: get sterilized bottle and milk, warm up bottle and feed baby as much as he'll take. Then get sterilized 50ml gastric syringe, surgical gloves, litmus paper, sterile water. Aspirate naso-gastric tube (i.e., draw back some fluid from the baby's gut, to check that the tube is indeed *in* the gut, not near the lungs – if it's become dislodged and you pour milk down it, you can drown the baby), and check the acidity of the fluid on the litmus paper. If satisfied, tube-feed remaining milk, then flush naso-gastric tube with sterile water. *Then* imagine having to be *compos mentis* enough to do all this at 3 a.m. – while trying not to wake sleeping husband. (Pete would do the 11 p.m. feed, to try and let me get to bed early, then go to bed himself; since he was back at work, I'd do all the wee small hours feeds.) It's amazing what you can get used to. And I even learned to 'pass' a naso-gastric tube – i.e. put it down the poor wee victim's gullet.

Outpatient appointments at Sick Kids produced
thumbs-up reports on his progress; he ate, slept, put on
weight, smiled, gurgled, and completely charmed the socks
off, *privatim et seriatim*,* health visitors, community nurses,
GPs, family, friends and chance-met strangers, and was
generally a good chap to have around. He finally started
to look and act more like a real person – and a wee cherub
to boot, particularly once he got rid of his naso-gastric
feeding tube – only a week or so before going south again
for the next op. His looks were at least briefly unmarred
by wire-work [i.e. the tube in his nose] – before it went
straight back in when the next procedures started. But at
least we got some photos of him without, to prove it!

Gill makes plain how the commitment to a child's medical needs
engulfs a whole family, siblings included. Gill's daughter had to join
the family's migration to her brother's bedside 200 miles away. At
two-and-a-half years old, she was keen to see him in ICU – and
then keen to leave quickly. Later in the ward, she tried to amuse
and cuddle him – not always practical while he was an in-patient
(and she was im-patient . . .). The family now laugh at how she
used to decorate him with her princess tiara as he sat in his little
seat. The aftermath of a 'stage 1' operation merges directly into the
preparation for 'stage 2,' so realistically to have a child born with
Hypoplastic Left Heart Syndrome takes a year out of everyone's
life. Ask Gill how they managed and she responds, 'Er . . .' The
question seems genuinely hard to answer. For her, considerations
of how the adults were coping seemed the very least important
part of the events of Michael's first year – and anyway they hadn't

---

* '*Privatim et seriatim*': privately and one after the other; a phrase loved by the
Victorians, who used it to describe the day's work of a prostitute, say, or the
interview engagements of a duke.

dared to think about this question for long periods. While they were in the eye of the hospital storm where crises were an everyday occurrence and while they were living alongside other hospital families that were falling apart under the stress, Gill and Pete simply clung together and rode the switchback – 'just tried to keep on keeping on, kept our fingers crossed and avoided analysing our own feelings'. After 'stage 2', the family came home 'feeling at first, sort of blank, and surprised; we *so* had trained ourselves to not plan beyond Op 2 – just in case – that we actually found it hard to pick up and *start* planning, and thinking what next, and make a future beyond a week or two. The weeks after getting home were some of the best times the family ever spent – just winding down slowly, and adjusting; finally feeling like proper family-life-with-two-kids has actually kick-started.'

Michael will remember nothing of all this. Most contemporary children are operated before they go to school, often while they are still babes in arms. One insightful child explained that it feels as if all the drama had happened to the 'little boy who was going to be me'. With no recall of the events, he cannot feel he is quite the same person as the mini-hero at the centre of some family myths and the photographs are perplexing and rather alarming to look at. If such a child is ever grateful for the life that his operation has given him, it is not because he remembers.

But many people who were older children at the time of their 'big operations' are bound to tell the stories of their own lives in a completely different way. The years after surgery are often keenly remembered for the new surge of vitality that they brought. It had been dispiriting for one sixteen-year-old to need another boy to run for him when he was batting at cricket; being barred from flying with the Air Force cadets had been crushing. But after the operation he became a 'completely different person'. Within a year, he was looping-the-loop with ex-Second World War pilots. The great novelty for a second boy was the possibility of going to a new school where the people around him did not know and could not guess that he had a cardiac problem. A third, who had his operation when he was nine, celebrated with BMX bikes and skateboards as he 'packed in about six years between the ages of ten and twelve. Suddenly there was a future.'

It might seem appealing to have the chance of 'being reborn', of getting a new start in life, but few of us would choose to go blind for the sake of experiencing the revelation of being able to see again. Similarly, nobody is reconsidering the policy of repairing children's hearts as early as is safe. It will be rare for future children to experience a transformative operation at an age when they are self-aware; they may grow up more 'normal', less 'special', and perhaps less grateful for life. We all want the good bits of others' lives but not the bad; the early patients who describe the euphoria of their newly found energy after their operations had paid for that experience with many years of slow-moving childhood. How can the memory of such a turnaround in your fortunes fail to influence your character?

13
Dirty washing

Not all homecomings are infused with optimism. Fearing this book would be a triumphalist account of the history of the treatment of congenital heart disease, one mother challenged me to include some not-so-good-news stories. I knew what she meant and all parents who have sat at an intensive care unit bed-side in any era know too; they have all felt dread. In a busy unit, a child will die most weeks. ICU parents wait together, drink coffee together, often share accommodation; and even families whose strategy has been to pull up the emotional drawbridges will know what is going on. But these stories are not about deaths.

Meet two young women, born in the 1980s and now both thirty-something. Both survived operations in early childhood and their hearts are tolerably well repaired. Helen is big and slow, with a sheepish curiosity and a small repertoire of conversation. She has a mental age of about three. Looking at her, you would know that Helen is 'different'. Not so Maria. She is pretty – though not always sweet – and passes at first as a normal young woman; she has the understanding capacity of a much younger child. Currently Helen lives happily in a little community with a team of guardians and a mini social life and Maria's carers know her well enough to get her cooperation and – on the surface – her lifestyle looks almost privileged. To arrive at this accommodation has taken an unenviable twenty-five years when each woman's family suffered the awful fallout of a short-lived medical crisis in the wards of two hospitals. Though their stories are in many ways similar, along the way their mothers made one decision differently.

Helen was born small and blue and her first hospital counselled her mother against pursuing treatment. After insisting that she at least be assessed, the more specialist unit recognized that Helen had Fallot's tetralogy, albeit at the bad end of the spectrum. Treatment would be available but it would be best if she could grow a bit. This took ages. Helen eventually learned to walk (more exactly she would walk, squat, walk) and was beginning to talk when she was called in for her surgery. It was a long operation but she eventually arrived back in the ICU. Her father went in to reconnoitre the situation and came back to his wife with news that their child was pink, awake and taking some notice of the world. Just as both parents were returning together, Helen had a cardiac arrest and when they next saw her she was limp and comatose. There followed a fortnight of intensive care before her mother got her first cuddle – of a floppy, unresponsive three-year-old who seemed to look around but not to see.*

Later, life at home was terrible – sleepless nights, lots of screaming. For years, Helen needed a buggy or wheelchair before she walked independently. Her vision improved, and at the age of eight she eventually started talking again. In term time a bus would collect her at 8.15 a.m. to go to a 'special' school, returning her at 4.15 p.m. – but in the long school holidays the family had to cope on their own. Home was depressed, claustrophobic and desperately lonely. Helen's father's refuge became his work, her mother's

---

* This is called 'cortical blindness'. The apparatus of the eye and nerve pathways work but the brain can't integrate the signals to reconstruct the image.

became Valium; paying for childcare was never an option. Teenage years were the worst, with a two-year-old in an adult body and a lot of tantrums. Helen's mother had more than one episode of 'failure to cope' when Helen's big sister had to step in and run the household – while trying to keep her own education going. With everyone at a low ebb, Helen's mother and a group of families of 'special needs' kids began a campaign for support and raised money that they used for occasional coach trips out of town. When school-days finished, there was no option of after-sixteen education. An interminable future stretched ahead. The local authority offered Helen's mother one day of 'respite care' every six weeks and an annual six-day break – though to make use of this, the family would have to book their holiday a year in advance. Getting help from the statutory authorities was a constant struggle until Helen was thirty-one, when she finally left home for a residential unit, living with other very dependent young adults and a rota of live-in carers. The state has taken over responsibility and Helen lives with friends and enjoys swimming once a week; the routine suits her limitations well and this has been by far the happiest time Helen or her mother have ever experienced. Her favourite video remains *Postman Pat*.

Maria is also a dependent young woman of thirty who lives in an annex to her mother's home. Besides her family, she has three paid carers. In addition, a personal trainer helps to keep her fit, a beautician comes to pluck her eyebrows, and every week she has an English lesson and a singing lesson. She has her own car, which her carers use to drive her about. She is hopeless with numbers and has no idea of time. At family gatherings, she tends to butt in and claim conversations. She can be rather rude and adversarial and – because she looks so normal – the public don't always tolerate her behaviour, leaving her family forever apologizing. Like Helen, this is by far the best period of life so far for both Maria and her mother, and this improvement is thanks to funding which provides her care package.

Getting Maria to these stable circumstances has not been easy. Her brain damage happened in the first month of her life. Blue at birth, Maria had a blocked pulmonary valve and a hole between the atria through which blood poured when it couldn't fight its way out to the lungs. She had a shunt on the third day of life and another at seven days. After the second operation, her mother overheard staff saying, 'Looks like a good job this time.' There followed months of Maria remaining blue and ill, before a third operation – this time a direct attack on the tight pulmonary valve itself – rendered her 'properly' pink. For a long time, Maria would not cooperate with feeding or even swallowing; her poor mother was desperate, often feeling that she was at war with her own toddler. Maria first walked when she was three and had a 'Statement of Special Educational Needs' by the time she entered primary school. On a clinic visit, her mother asked the cardiologist if congenital heart disease and learning difficulties went hand in hand, but the answer came back 'No'. She contacted a barrister friend who suggested that she approach the hospital more formally, but their response after reviewing the notes was that 'Nothing untoward had happened'. Maria's father left home. Maria herself grew to be a very self-centred, unsettled, anxious little girl whose behaviour could make life a nightmare for the people around her.

The next event was a high-profile television documentary reporting an anaesthetist's claim that the care of infants in their particular hospital was sub-standard. The whistleblower later returned to Australia, but his claims eventually triggered a full public inquiry into the children's heart services of Maria's hospital. Maria's case was one of many that were reviewed and the story her mother told contributed in some part to her particular surgeons being barred from operating and to the breaking-down of the 'club culture' that had developed between the clinicians and the hospital management to draw a veil over the poor performance of the cardiac team. Litigation in the High Court followed, and Maria's case was the

first to be heard. From its initiation to settlement, this took twelve
years. It is the financial compensation that has made Maria's present life relatively comfortable – but it did not arrive until she was
in her mid twenties. Similar to the experiences of Helen's family,
the struggles of schooling and adolescence had been unrelenting.
One after another, state-system schools and private-sector schools
had failed to cope with Maria's conduct. Her mother learned that
getting into a special needs unit was harder than getting into Eton.
There were constant phone calls and demands on her mother from
school administrations that could not cope with Maria's combative
behaviour. In her teenage years, all the stress triggered a breakdown,
with Maria hallucinating, pacing and inaccessible to human contact.
During the darkest period, a policeman, a psychiatrist and a social
worker took her away to a closed mental hospital where she was
detained under the Mental Health Act. In the aftermath of this, the
local authority at last stepped in with what they called a 'care package' and, in the longer run, natural maturity has gradually helped.

No two cases of brain damage are the same either in their
cause or their effect. When a parent gives consent to any cardiac
operation, the possibility of brain damage will be mentioned in the
small print; this acknowledges the reality that we still do not know
everything about protecting brains in heart surgery and its aftermath, and even if every reasonable precaution is taken, problems
can develop. Individuals and families experiencing these inexplicable complications have only the support of their own relatives and
whatever publicly funded provisions are offered. However, if it can
be demonstrated *both* that the damage would not have occurred
had a 'reasonably competent medical professional' undertaken the
procedure *and* that the 'injury resulted as a direct result of the negligent action', there may be the basis for a legal claim for financial
compensation.

We do not know if Helen's damage was the result of medical negligence, though if the underlying cause was air in her

bloodstream, which can cause both cardiac arrest and brain damage, this is quite likely. Her mother did consider pursuing the issue, but decided against it, reckoning correctly that it would have been a hard and lonely path. The family had put their trust in the unit where she was operated, and in the doomed atmosphere after Helen's prolonged coma there had even been a party when a neighbour who had run a marathon had presented a cheque to the ward. Something told Helen's mother that litigation 'just wasn't done'. Maria's mother took the opposite line. The public inquiry had aired some of the 'dirty washing' of the unit where her daughter had been operated and this had chimed with her personal impressions of the team. Though she was never part of its publicly vociferous fringe, Maria's mother knew that other parents were prepared to take on the system. Left with an irretrievably damaged child of ten years of age, Maria's mother already understood that 'there is no justice'. Bitterness or retribution were also futile and she has never indulged these thoughts. It was funding and the choices it could provide for the future that was at stake.

The process was hard: twelve years of paperwork, meetings and waiting for the post to arrive, trying not to lose faith. The trial process itself was painful. During the proceedings, she sat next to the very surgeon whose professionalism was in question and watched him doing a crossword puzzle. Once the negligence of the hospital had been determined, the amount of financial compensation to be awarded became the main issue. It was clear that Maria would never work and 'loss of earnings' was part of the quantum. The defence barristers tried to minimize what Maria's earning potential might have been with the implication that her mother 'only worked in catering' – difficult to listen to for a graduate who helped run the family business. On the other hand, Maria's examination by an independent neurologist whose task it was to document the scale of the brain damage proved a useful encounter. It was bizarre for Maria's mother to hear the specialist

'read' her daughter's personality problems from her brain scan. 'The
frontal lobe damage would deprive her of empathy, she would be
abrupt and rude, sometimes narcissistic, a poor planner.' These were
'hardwired' but could be worked around. 'Reward good behaviour,
ignore the bad.' 'It might be a good idea to keep some education
going well into adult life.' This was the first authoritative, person-
alized advice about managing Maria's particular difficulties that
her mother had ever received. She lost her embarrassment about her
daughter's behaviour in public – nothing could be done, it was
not her fault. The reports were submitted, the defence appealed,
but eventually the settlement came in and was generous enough
to fund the 'princess' lifestyle that now suits Maria so well. With
Maria happier, everyone is happier. Her mother submits some
paperwork annually documenting the outgoings – a huge change
from the years confronting the bureaucracy of claiming statutory
provisions. Her mother is the first to say that the legal route was
a severe endurance test; she could not afford to lose momentum
for more than a couple of months over twelve years. But she was a
starter-finisher by temperament – one of those people who say they
will run a marathon and actually do it – and she is quietly proud of
persevering with the battle. That said, she is daily reminded of what
has clearly been taken away from her daughter – independence and
opportunities to move on with her life. For Maria, the best possible
way of spending an evening is to be curled up on the sofa with
one of her carers, watching *X-Factor* with a TV dinner on her lap.

   The Bristol Royal Infirmary Inquiry reported in 2001 after
being in the national headlines for months. It listed almost 200 recommendations for improvement of the Bristol service in particular,
the conduct of paediatric cardiac services generally and also for
the whole British National Health Service. It shook the specialty
in the UK, most doctors and specialist units quietly realizing that
'there but for fortune' one or other of the criticisms could easily
have come their way. The damning claim was that between 1991

and 1995, thirty to thirty-five children undergoing heart surgery at Bristol Royal Infirmary had died who would probably have survived if they had been treated elsewhere. The statistical techniques that backed this claim have been integrated into a rolling audit of surgical outcomes; these are available to the public. For many reasons, mortality for infant surgery has dropped since the beginning of this century, and most professionals in the field would agree that this is due in part to more transparency. That said, a shunt such as the one Maria received as a newborn baby remains one of the highest-risk operations in a cardiac surgeon's repertoire – and would be an unusual approach in tackling pulmonary stenosis today. But Maria was logged as a survivor and even now – more than fifteen years after the inquiry reported – there would be no acknowledgement in the official statistics of the scale of brain damage experienced by either Maria or Helen, or of the toll on their families, or even any credible evidence about whether the incidence of such major damage is falling or rising.

The furore about Bristol was widely reported and some parents of children who had died there were bitterly vocal in the criticism of the surgeons in particular. But for other families – Richard's, for example – this condemnation was very hard to listen to. The surgeon most criticized had changed Richard's life. Before his operation, he had been a thirteen-year-old schoolboy who was so restricted that he was delegated to fold up the team's football kit indoors while his friends actually went out to play. In hospital, this very surgeon had talked Richard through the operation, giving him great confidence. The outcome had been excellent and he was soon trekking with the Boy Scouts. In gratitude, a few years later he sent his surgeon what we now call a 'selfie' from the top of Ben Nevis. When the Bristol Heart Service controversies hit the news, the stories were so painful that Richard's parents simply refused to believe them; they had trusted their precious son to the hands of this surgeon. At first, Richard himself followed the press, cutting articles out of *Private Eye* and the national papers – but at some stage he too realized that he did not want to know any more and tore them all up. Losing trust is so painful – as in a marriage when a partner does not want to believe some malicious gossip. Years later, a cardiologist reviewing Richard said, 'Say what you like about Wisheart, he did a good job on you.'

14
Flying solo

'The sword of Gryffindor was hidden they knew not where, and they were three teenagers in a tent whose only achievement was not, yet, to be dead.'
    – J. K. Rowling, *Harry Potter and the Deathly Hallows*

For this venture I have talked to teenagers, but completely candid conversations are difficult. For them, I am too old; there is too much to explain. Anyway, perhaps it is no fairer to generalize about teenagers with congenital heart disease than it is to make sweeping statements about teenagers at all. So I need to fall back on my own experience of 'adolescent' patients, with all its subjectivity. In the spirit of full disclosure, I should therefore declare how much respect I have for many of them. Like Harry Potter and his friends, they have already proved something by simply being alive, but some still have thoughts of the 'Deathly Hallows' they need to come to terms with.

Except that many really do not (face an evil foe). For some diagnoses, we have had enough patients through the world's hospitals to know that they pretty much merge with their contemporaries in terms of their chance of a long life. Whether anyone has ever spelled this out to the young people themselves is another matter. All through their childhoods they attend hospital clinics, often only picking up cryptic information that was pitched at their parents. At the very least, and unlike most of their friends, a teen-ager with a scar on their chest may not feel indestructible.

Frequent hospital trips connect some children's whole upbring-ings with the uncertainty of life, yet many seem to appreciate that their very survival accentuates their own vitality. Though they may not even remember their operations, they have understood that coming through them is a great achievement, shared with their doctors, their parents and their own bodies. For them, it was not a matter of heroism but of some sort of core strength. Perhaps I am fanciful, but I sense that some of these young people have a 'certain something'.

I also recognize some whose tests show they are quite restricted after palliative operations and whose future I would be guarded about, but who seem very committed to living. They do well at college and seem to have an enthusiasm for social life, thriving on the usual vigorous regime of phone messaging. When I inquire, they report no problems. If they are 'in denial', it seems an effect-ive strategy.

Still others sit mute in the clinic while their parents are ready with stories of achievement and family solidarity – though I some-times sense that their 'heart warrior' narrative sits uncomfortably with the young person himself; I cannot be sure. I do know that a few have laid into their parents for not letting them die as babies rather than putting them through so much 'for so little' – painful for everybody, but adolescents punishing their parents is not so rare. A few seem to use their hearts as a get-out clause that permits them not to try anything too difficult. In fairness, some modern operations are 'miracles' in offering children a life at all, but not 'miracles' in providing a life like everyone else's. It is one thing to be 'special', but most teenagers want to be 'special' in exactly the same way their friends are.

To unpack my question about what makes young people's attitudes seem so diverse after apparently similar medical experiences,
I approached Liza. Liza has 'dual nationality'; she is a psychologist
who is also a patient who can map her personal history by the many
scars on her own body; through a support group, she also speaks
to many others. She resists my suggestion that there is one set of
people who respond negatively to traumatic events and another
set who experience personal growth; it is too simplistic, we jump
too easily to conclusions. We humans make great efforts to project
ourselves to others, making it difficult to notice the hurt behind
one individual's stoicism or the core resilience behind another's
apparent distress.

As our conversation goes on, I am made to realize how we
adults take the view that situations that would be considered
traumatic for a child in any other walk of life are assumed to be
benevolent when they occur in a medical setting and in the name
of saving their life. The corresponding child's-eye view of their
situation is not necessarily benign. Is what they experience in hospital so different from physical abuse – the pain, the occasional
pin-downs, even the warning of the 'punishment' to come? The
grown-ups (doctors and family members) collude with this paradox
as a cushion for *themselves* as they observe a child's physical ordeal.
Though it is an even more uncomfortable thought, childhood
experiences of recurrent hospital exposures also have uneasy simi-
larities to the humiliations of childhood sexual abuse – undressing
for strangers, wandering hands, invasion of body-boundaries, lack
of control, issues of trust and distrust, the obligatory silence, dis-
sociation, flashbacks . . .

Liza observes how patients are even nudged to feel grateful
for it all. She says, 'Although I feel immensely grateful, under
these circumstances, this gratitude is frequently the only acceptable
emotion.' The children are left cornered in the role their supporters
want them to play, coping in their heads as they try to reconcile

the messages they are receiving from their bodies with the picture described by their doctors and family. It is so easy to ask children to air their anxieties and then offer them nothing but reassurance. Reassurance is the fastest way for adults to close the conversation down when they feel under pressure; someone called 'premature reassurance' the 'roadblock to listening'. Heart children will have heard a lot of that. No wonder some teenagers are resentful.

★ ★ ★

Of all the patients who have had a childhood operation, some will eventually get a 'You are good to go' appraisal – like the 'All clear, we don't need to see you again' that people hope for after cancer treatment. Some who are completely well after a straightforward operation such as an atrial or ventricular septal defect closure or treatment for not-too-severe blockage at their pulmonary valve may at some time receive this happy news. Free from any pressure to return to hospital clinics, they are launched into their futures just like everyone else – with only a scar and a backstory to go with it.

Currently, this happens to rather less than half the people operated on in childhood. For the rest, some concern keeps them on the books of specialists – concern either that their heart is already less than good or uncertainty that it may become less than 'good enough' in the future. These people are asked to return periodically for check-ups for the rest of their lives and some are told to expect further surgery. They cannot leave the problem behind. Nevertheless, by the time they hit teenage life, most congenital heart patients will have had their major operation. Surgery will have delivered all it can offer for the moment and the young person needs to get on as best they can with whatever has been achieved. Whether they merge completely with the crowd or stand apart in some way depends only partly on the state of their hearts.

★ ★ ★

Mostly, after their 'big' operations children, teenagers and adults are pink (or almost pink) and not obviously disabled or different. Most patients manage most everyday things, and in practice nobody notices if someone never seems to run up the stairs. This means that there is no conversation to be had about a heart history unless the person affected brings up the subject – or unless somebody sees their scar and curiosity sparks questions. It is hard to avoid a stranger glimpsing a scar and wanting to know how it came about, but most patients have perfected a quick comeback to deflect too much curiosity – one boy got away with 'I was attacked by a shark' for several years.

These days there are some valve interventions that can be done in the X-ray department which do not leave a mark and we are at the beginning of being able to do more radical 'keyhole surgery' on the heart. But for the present, a scar is the badge that almost all cardiac survivors wear, and it is often the scar that provokes the inquisitive. Just where a scar lies depends on the particular operation and the surgical fashions at the time. Mickey Shaw and other survivors from open-heart operations of the 1950s typically had huge incisions from armpit to armpit; the breastbone was cut horizontally with bone-cutting shears. This must have been tremendously painful in the subsequent weeks, but once the tissues have knitted together these scars are easily kept secret, even with an open necked shirt or under a bikini top. Some parts of the heart or circulation can be reached by smaller horizontal incisions between the ribs on one or other side of the chest – serving for shunts, repairs on narrow aortas (coarctation) or high-pressure lung arteries (banding), and a few open-heart procedures. The scars these operations leave are also easily hidden, even under skimpy clothes, though some girls did have later problems: as they grew up, it transpired that the incisions made when they were little had gone through their immature breast tissue and after puberty this resulted in very lopsided development. Surgery can improve this – though the operation may need more planning than comes naturally to some cosmetic surgeons.*

Most open-heart operations these days are done through what is called a 'median sternotomy' – a cut right down the middle of the chest, the breastbone being split along its length with a power saw. The aesthetics of the resulting scar depend partly on the age of the child; the older you are the uglier the scar you can expect – tiny babies heal beautifully (and surgery on a fetus leaves barely any mark). Conversely, some people have an unfortunate tendency to make strong but very lumpy scars called keloids; this propensity is probably genetic and people of African heritage are especially prone to it. The surgeon and the sewing thread he uses are important too; again his choices were influenced by the date. Nowadays most surgeons take pride in stitching up an incision as though it had never been there. The fine filament suture material is sewn underneath the skin and gradually dissolves so there are no stitches to take out; at their best, these leave a neat white line. Not so in the 1960s, when children would be given little jars to take home containing their big black sutures with their spidery knots; those stitches left their marks.

Having said all that, people's attitude to their scars does not seem to depend primarily on the cosmetic result, more on what it means. For children needing a series of operations, their scars are like a map of their lives. At best many find them a poignant personal reminder that they were once very vulnerable and at worst (a quarter in one survey) patients positively dislike or hate their scar. Though the body-fascism of adolescence can be a real challenge for children who are not at ease with their scars, most can choose

---

* Both the women I spoke to who had had cosmetic breast surgery had complications because their plastic surgeons had treated them just like any other breast augmentation patient – for example 'forgetting' that they were on anticoagulants.

to hide them in everyday life; but if you look 'normal' with your winter clothes on, when summer comes, do you dress to conceal your scar? Bernhard, born in 1948 and with both shunt and repair scars, didn't even recognize the question: 'I never thought about it, never talked about it, even to my wife. Perhaps men are more shallow like that.' Gemma, born in 1979 and petite with sternotomy, pacemaker and abdominal scars, wears a bikini with unflagging pride; if people stare she asks, 'Would you like to take a photo?'* A few patients have even accentuated their scars with astonishing tattoos – perhaps an ECG trace that helps them tell their story.

But for many people, showing their scar is a 'coming out' decision. Most patients are very cautious about who they tell – and give good reasons for their reticence. It is not that they are being deceitful but many feel safer 'in the closet'. Because of occasional bad experiences, many have become cautious about who they can trust. Can 'we' be counted on not to overreact? Patients say that 'we' are prone to labelling them as either 'warriors' or as 'losers' – both absurd stereotypes. Can 'we' be trusted not to kick them out of the team because of our *own* anxieties about their reliability? (Patients worry about exclusion and 'career suicide': in our ignorance, might we marginalize them on the pretext of 'risk management' or 'precaution'?) Can we be trusted not to gossip? (Like most privacy issues, people like a sense of control over health-related information.) Many adult patients can count on their fingers the number of people who know about their heart history. Yet it would all be a whole lot easier for people with scars on their chests if we were more aware that they are already around us, working away in our midst!

---

* This is exactly what a Scottish support group did, producing 'Scarred for Life', a photo-journalistic exhibition of people showing and talking about their scars. http://www.thesf.org.uk/campaigning-for-you/scarred-for-life.aspx

At every turning point in their lives, people can – and do – change their minds about who to tell; when they enter a new school, college or job, move to a new neighbourhood or start a new relationship. But there comes a time in a person's life story when they need to share what they know with someone intimate, and this usually involves talking about what the scar means for the future as well as the past. For patients operated in the early days, these were especially difficult conversations. There were no truthful answers – they were the first people in the history of the planet ever to survive with congenital heart disease and there was no map for their futures.

★   ★   ★

Before surgery was available, hardly anyone born with a condition of any complexity survived to adolescence. Even the very first wave of surgery arguably produced only 'elite survivors' – patients whose original anatomy was particularly favourable and who were lucky enough to get a really good repair; the rest simply died at operation.

There are currently more young people than ever whose teenage years are compromised in some way by their hearts. Nowadays babies born with malformations that cannot ever be reorganized into something resembling a normal heart undergo a series of operations that will allow them at least to stay alive. Though each individual operation is risky, in practice most do now make it through. Perhaps they have tubes or valves implanted that will need replacing as they grow. Perhaps they are left with one pumping chamber instead of two. For such operations, there is a phrase – 'definitive palliation' – to identify the final operation.[*]

---

[*] Definitive palliations involving tubes (that a child may grow out of) include repair of Truncus Arteriosus and Rastelli operations. No operation that involves replacing a valve can be thought of as 'forever' – and don't let us forget that transplantation is palliative too.

The Fontan operation (see page 226) and its lookalikes (e.g. Total Cavo Pulmonary Connection) are the 'definitive palliations' for all hearts with only one good ventricle (their 'stage 3'). They share the principle that the blue blood returning to the heart is diverted directly into the lungs without the benefit of a pumping ventricle. This leaves the single good ventricle to serve the body. It's the best we can do. We are doing more 'definitive palliations' than ever before – the Fontan procedure is now the commonest operation in children over the age of two.

Under ideal circumstances, most of these 'fixes' work quite well – the patients look pink, though their hearts cannot usually boost their output on exercise as much as the patients would like. Teenagers with these 'definitive palliatiation' operations can literally get left behind – their mates move fast. In short, though many teenagers with scars join the mainstream of life, there remain some with secret and not-so-secret struggles.

A teenager in the 1990s, Christine had complex pulmonary atresia and despite two operations to reorganize the very exotic routes taken by the blood to reach her lungs, no inside-the-heart repair had been possible and she was still blue. Her school site had lifts but they were reserved for students in wheelchairs. A learning-support assistant would carry her bag between lessons – 'embarrassing or what?' Someone was delegated to look out for her on school trips because she got breathless. Other teachers 'forgot' and sent her out to (fail to) play netball in the rain. She had a couple of good friends and some academic strengths, but an 'ordinary teenage life' – if that exists – was not really available. And throughout all this time she wanted so much to be normal.

Rules about mandatory sports participation vary between schools, but I have heard stories of martinet sports teachers from everywhere. Paul was born in 1967 with Truncus Arteriosus, the 'trunk' being a lone artery coming out of the heart and branching to supply both the body and the lungs. In 1967, nobody had come up with a fix for this situation, but in response to his mother's refusal to 'let him go' surgeons put 'bands' around the two lung vessels to limit the flow through them and protect the vessels beyond from damage. This was done in the hope that Paul might survive until someone came up with a long-term solution, and in 1975 he did have a 'definitive palliation' that involved putting an external tube between the heart and the lung arteries. His early childhood had been very protected and he had learned to 'keep low, don't be noticed', but by adolescence he desperately wanted to merge. His PE teacher would call anyone not wearing shorts in the snow a 'sissy' and would have much preferred Paul to stay indoors, out of sight and out of mind. But for Paul the least-worst choice was to go out with the others, wearing a tracksuit and taking the flak.

Even now there are still Christines and Pauls negotiating teenage life with modified but not corrected hearts, though improvements in surgery have meant that hardly any are wheelchair-bound. Also, since the beginning of children's heart surgery, educational policies and disability legislation have both moved on. The Civil Rights movements of the 1960s in the USA produced laws that prohibited discrimination on the grounds of race or sex, but still did not embrace the rights of disabled people.* In England too, Race Relations and Equal Pay Acts both predated any attention to society's responsibilities towards children or adults with disabilities. But since the mid 1970s, on both sides of the Atlantic, there has been gradual progress at integrating the physically less able into the mainstream. In slightly different terms around the world, legislation

* Indeed the last 'Ugly Law' in the USA was only repealed in 1971. It required that 'No person who is diseased, maimed, mutilated or in any way deformed so as to be an unsightly or disgusting object or improper person to be allowed in or on the public ways or other public places in this city, or shall therein or thereon expose himself to public view, under a penalty of not less than one dollar nor more than fifty dollars for each offense.'

now specifies that a person with a disability should not receive less favourable treatment simply on account of their disability, and that 'reasonable adjustments' should be made to school and working environments to accommodate people like Christine and Paul. Unfortunately, as any parent will tell you, getting the law right is only the beginning of the story.

★   ★   ★

Though they may look back with exasperation at how ignorant individuals might try to sabotage them, most patients say that life with a health problem is largely what you make of it – and it is in our teenage years when we really begin to write our own life-scripts. Two young men, each with only one functioning ventricle, recounted how they had taken themselves in hand. James is the first to say that confidence was his issue. He was in his late teenage years before his Fontan plumbing and heart rhythms were really optimized – still 'not great' but as good as they were going to get. Then he took charge of his own attitude and the rest of his body. He realized that he was too skinny and made efforts to put on weight and muscle. The exercise regime to which he committed himself was very daunting at first – he would vomit after exertion – but he persevered and gradually improved to the extent that he could play one set of tennis.

The second young man was Tom, with whom I got in touch after seeing a photograph. He is a recently qualified doctor and even when we 'met' on Skype, I could see that he was tall, dark and handsome. The photograph that had caught my eye had shown him as a medical student towering over the other surgeons as he assisted at a Norwood operation – the operation he had undergone himself for his own Hypoplastic Left Heart condition more than two decades earlier. By his own account, in his early adolescence he had used his heart condition as a pretext for not really trying – or as an excuse for not succeeding – at 'stuff'. So what had turned that around? 'Attending "Camp del Corazon"'* with so many other kids with congenital heart problems was an eye-opening experience that showed me that I had to stop expecting sympathy from others and that I had to take control of my future. I realized that I could instead use my heart-history to motivate myself to become anything or anybody I wanted to.'

These guys were impressive, but I most enjoyed listening to four women in their fifties as they looked back on their adolescence, their common theme being how they had managed somehow to be 'normal' despite their manifest health difficulties. Judith was still a bit under par despite two operations for an Atrioventricular Septal Defect,† but as a 1970s teenager she babysat for the children next door and on her fifteenth birthday got herself a proper haircut, had her ears pierced and felt completely grown-up and normal. She met her 'first boys' at an Air Force cadets rock and roll disco but her first date was trumped by having to go into hospital for her 'first mitral valve replacement'. What teenager would want that? But she did bounce back.

In a different English small town, Jo was tiny and a bit blue; she had been born with only one good ventricle in the era before Fontan surgery and the two operations aimed at giving her not too little but not too much lung-blood flow‡ remain all the surgery she has had to date at the age of fifty. At weekends, she would buy a pizza with

---

* A summer camp on an island off the Californian coast, organized for children with heart disease by a non-profit organization and staffed by volunteers.
† This is a hole right in the middle of the heart. The bottom of the atria septum is involved as well as the ventricular septum, and because this is the area where the mitral and tricuspid valves are anchored, these have often formed abnormally.
‡ A Glenn operation and a Brock operation. In Jo's Glenn operation, the superior caval vein was chopped off the right atrium and the right pulmonary artery off the main pulmonary artery. The vessels were then sewn together so that all the blue blood returning from the upper body has nowhere else to go but into the right lung. In a Brock operation a metal instrument is poked through the

her pals and sit on the bench outside the library gossiping; when the time came, she smoked and drank with the rest of them.

Sandra had operations on her aortic valve as a baby and her mitral valve as a child – and others since. She was 'very naughty', loved clubbing and got pregnant when she was sixteen. Her cardiologist, who had looked out for her since early childhood, shouted at her in the outpatient clinic, 'Get in my room NOW.' Sandra was scared of her, but held her ground; she miscarried, but quickly got pregnant again and now has eight grandchildren. (When I asked her cardiologist about Sandra, she rolled her eyes and agreed that she had been a 'very naughty girl' – after fifty years, they are still in touch.)

Marilyn was a teenager in Los Angeles. Still blue with her Fallot's tetralogy uncorrected, she and her friends met 'three guys in a '57 Chevy'. The subsequent storyline involved mistaken phone numbers and would make a plot for a Hollywood movie, but she had met her future husband. I am in awe of these women, who seem to have had a lot more adolescent fun than I ever had with my tame long-term view of life.

★   ★   ★

Drifting away from parental control is the first joy of adolescence, but it throws up personal responsibilities too. Depending on the jurisdiction, sometime in teenage life the law turns you into an adult. At this point, a young person is deemed able to sign their own paperwork for surgery. In the USA, a parent signs these forms until their child is eighteen years of age (unless they are 'emancipated' – meaning that they are married, have a child or are in the military). In Britain, a young person can sign for themselves, even in defiance of their parents under some circumstances. Anywhere between the ages of sixteen and eighteen, refereeing

wall of the right ventricle and up into the pulmonary artery, the surgeon guiding it from the outside with his fingers. It will help forward flow from heart to lung.

decision-making between parent, child and doctor can be a delicate matter. It is hard to force an operation on a sixteen-year-old, even when their parents want it to proceed, and conversely a young person may request an operation that their parents reject, provided the doctors are on their side. Sophie's story is an example of the first scenario and Susie's of the second.

Sophie was born with Fallot's tetralogy, needed a shunt in the first month of life and was repaired when she was two – treatment typical of the early 1990s. Though she had no symptoms, by the time she was twelve years old the doctors had noticed that her lung arteries were not growing well and tests began to show that a lot of blood being pumped out by her right heart was simply sloshing backwards into the ventricle again. Solemn conversations began about the timing of another operation to sort out the narrowing and to put in a valve to stop the leak. After discussion, it was agreed that it might be best to schedule the surgery to minimize the effect on Sophie's exam preparation. The problem was that these negotiations had been between doctors and parents; fifteen-year-old Sophie was kept out of the loop.

She did not know that an operation was planned until a hospital visit just beforehand; she was not pleased. She felt well, she felt angry and in all honesty, she felt scared. Her parents delivered her to the hospital, but by the time she was due to go down for her operation she had realized that her parents had known for months, had signed all the forms and had not mentioned anything to her. They had treated her like a baby; she was beyond furious. A hopeful anaesthetist tried to persuade her to take a tablet – 'just a painkiller' – but she understood the ruse immediately and absolutely refused to cooperate at all. The staff capitulated and sent her home.

She returned two weeks later, still very cross and barely talking to her parents. The operation to do some 'cosmetic' surgery on her lung arteries and to put in a pulmonary valve went smoothly and she was home five days later. But the breach of trust with her parents still rankles ten years later. She now knows that her doctor had offered to talk to her about the operation, but her parents had declined. Sophie readily admits that – had she been consulted – she would probably have refused surgery, and probably her parents had intuited this. Now ten years older, she realizes there was fear as well as anger; without death ever being mentioned, it was clearly at least possible that she could die during the operation. On reflection, an explicit conversation might not have helped much: 'a teenager doesn't know the difference between "possible" and "really, really unlikely"' – but they do hate being patronized.

Contrast Sophie's lack of enthusiasm with Susie's predicament. Susie had received a shunt for pulmonary atresia when she was three months old. From the age of nine, she remembers the gist of clinic conversations being that if she did not get another operation she would die before she was twenty. At some stage in her teens an operation seemed to have been agreed between her mother and the doctors, but months passed with no news; in retrospect her mother was probably declining admission dates. On the one occasion Susie did go in to hospital, her mother removed her again without explanation. It could not have been clearer that her mother did not want surgery to go ahead; still nobody consulted Susie. The family atmosphere deteriorated to the extent that Susie left home for a while. When she was seventeen, a clinic doctor contrived to peel her away from her mother and explained that she was old enough to commit to the operation for herself. She agreed, honestly thinking that she would die – that was what had been instilled in her; that was her 'destiny'. She signed, submitted and survived. It took a couple of years to realign her sense of having a future. Much later, her mother explained that she had felt 'like a lioness rejecting its weakest cub'; mother and daughter have never really mended their relationship.

★   ★   ★

The 'coming of age' in the legal sense is paralleled by another transition in most medical services dealing with teenagers. At some stage, the team of paediatricians, nurses and children's wards that have often been looking after them from birth must say 'good-bye'. Whether or not there is a 'hello' from a corresponding team competent to deal with adults with scars from congenital heart operations depends on time and place. Now that the numbers of adults with congenital heart disease far exceed the numbers of children, it seems unthinkable that specialist services to look after those people have not always been in place. In fact they were very much needed long before they existed.

Before 1960, there were few adult survivors of congenital heart disease because surgery was effectively rationed by the 'lottery' of access to treatment. A lack of awareness on the part of non-specialists and their subsequent failure to refer meant that not all children who would have benefited actually got an operation. Also surgical facilities were few. During the 1960s, the number of specialist centres grew and began to match the demand – and patients were beginning to survive in impressive numbers. But if the doctors of that time told those patients how they were going to get on in life, they were bluffing – there was no evidence to go on.

One problem was over-optimism. Surgeons would claim to have 'corrected' defects when actually they had often left old problems behind and created new ones. Perhaps imperfect valves were left untouched because they were not the pressing issue at the time of operation, though years later the valve's shortcomings would impact the heart and thus the patient. Surgery also leaves 'internal' scars behind – you cannot cut into heart muscle without impairing its contraction or its strength or its electrical excitability. But complications related to any of these shortcomings can take time to declare themselves, so an operated youngster may have 'fled the nest' of his childhood hospital before troubles arise.

Another obstacle was a lack of humility on the part of cardiologists. Before around 1980, if a teenager was to be followed up at all, it had to be by an adult cardiologist whose bread and butter would be earned from looking after much older patients with rheumatic heart disease or coronary artery disease. For such doctors, their rare patients who had undergone congenital heart operations were very exotic. Many patients remember being paraded in front of medical students, the senior doctor showing off as the novices stumbled through the physical examination and failed to make sense of all the clues as to what was wrong. Some of those cardiologists made no attempt to keep up with the fast-moving world of congenital heart medicine yet were loath to refer 'their' patients to the few who did.

What needed to happen was some acknowledgement of the uncertain futures that these patients faced and for plans to be made to keep systematic track of them. Some patients who had no long-term follow-up arrangements before around 1980 have still not returned to clinics and others who thought they were cured began to experience problems that nobody diagnosed. Because the patients were so dispersed, if a lone patient ran into problems, he was managed by a lone doctor who worked by trial and error; this is no way to advance medical understanding. Doctors have some sort of medical instinct to say, 'Don't worry' when the symptoms that a patient suffers and the findings on examination do not fit a pattern that they recognize. It is a difficult cultural problem and addressing it requires some humility on the doctor's part – which doesn't always come.

The first place where any authoritative service for adults with congenital heart disease emerged was in London. Just as Helen Taussig had put the specialty of congenital heart disease on the map, Jane Somerville – another inconvenient female doctor who breached the glass ceiling of the male-dominated mainstream – did the same for the specialty that came to be called 'Grown-Up-Congenital Heart' disease (GUCH or now ACHD,

Adult-CHD). Dr Somerville had learned cardiac surgery, paediatric cardiology and adult cardiology in the services of the foremost specialists in the country. She knew from her apprenticeship in operating rooms that very few operations were as 'corrective' as advertised. Appointed as an adult cardiologist, she set up a ward for children and young adults in 1975, and points to the World Congress of Paediatric Cardiology in 1980 as being the inception of the ACHD speciality. From around that time, the medical community began to acknowledge the merits of collecting patients together and of formally training young doctors in what was rapidly becoming a brand-new branch of medicine.

As arrangements currently exist, most young people 'graduate' to adult services at around the age of sixteen. Many find their first clinic appointment after 'transition' intimidating; it is often their first experience of attending hospital without a parent. They may be asked quite pertinent questions about their medical past – and perhaps they cannot answer accurately. The realization dawns that they need to know – what if they were taken to an emergency department after an accident and asked about what operation their scar represented, what would they say? In other ways, these first clinics without parents hanging around can be welcome – a chance to have grown-up conversations about contraception (how many other adolescents get the chance to do that?) or to ask direct questions about their futures without upsetting their families.

★   ★   ★

For most doctors working at the childhood end of the specialty, the last appointment before a child moves to a transition clinic is a happy/sad moment – relief that you have delivered them to a future, but also a goodbye because you will probably never hear of them again. Information travels forwards with the patient, but news does not necessarily come 'backwards' from their future lives. Childhood doctors may hear back from the adult services to which they sent their patients, but the information comes as statistics – perhaps the numbers of patients in different diagnostic categories who die or are reoperated. All the names are stripped out, so the continuity of the relationship is lost.

Except sometimes. Doctors do have favourite patients (actually I have several). I don't care too much for pretty hearts – give me someone who has been through some shit. Often my favourites are young people who – I hope – have taught me something important.

As a trainee, I held a retractor during Stephen's original surgery. He must have been about two years old and we knew at the time that the operation was compromised – the hole in his ventricular septum was hard to reach, hard to close. I met him again when he was about six years old and I had almost finished my training as a paediatric cardiologist. Later, as his consultant, I sent him to his second repair. He showed off his break-dance moves in the clinic when he was about twelve and at the peak of his physical capacity. He grew tall, black and beautiful, would later turn up alone to clinics, in his school uniform, unbooked, if he wanted a chat. He was the only seriously cool person who has ever given me the time of day. Once he asked me whether or not he would live long enough to get through medical school. 'Maybe not.' He wanted me to promise not to let his mother know. 'Okay, unless she asks.' By the time he transferred to adult services he was losing ground. We kept in touch. He threw himself into making thoughtful films and living hard. One night, he collapsed at a disco and was resuscitated by his friends, but the ventilator was switched off weeks later when his mother finally accepted that he was not coming back.

15
Grown up and trying to do normal things

With no predecessors to learn from, the earliest survivors of congenital heart surgery grew up without any road-map for their lives. They did not know in advance if it was realistic to expect to do normal things – work, marry, have babies or bury their own parents.

Most of the adults who have helped with this book have jobs. They include: anaesthetist, artist, bass guitarist, café manager, carpenter, computer programmer, drummer, children's nurse, clerical officer, dentist, father, graphic designer, hairdresser, human resources manager, librarian, mother, nurse, priest, psychiatric nurse, psychotherapist, psychologist, receptionist, security guard, semi-professional footballer, shipwright, social worker, solicitor, store manager, Storm Trooper (sadly only as a film extra), student, teacher, telephone operative, unemployed, university administrator. If you know anyone doing one of these jobs, they might be hiding a childhood scar under their clothes and – just as Clark Kent conceals his Superman outfit under his city suit – you might never realize.

For most people, being in work matters; employment brings an income and is central to many people's identity and role in society.

Arguably my informants are particularly obliging people so their spectrum of jobs is perhaps not representative; perhaps their very willingness to help me makes them too exceptional to be typical of all 'graduates' of childhood heart surgery. A few formal surveys exist researching the proportion of adults with congenital heart disease who are employed. In one British review, compared to their same-sex peers, the surveyed patients were five times more likely to have been out of work for more than a year. It would be simple to pin the shortfall in employment on the seriousness of the heart problems these people were born with, or on the incompleteness of their surgical repairs, but this turns out to be too simplistic. Unless a person's health is very poor, the statistics suggest that there is little correlation between a patient's cardiac wellbeing and their capacity either to work or to enjoy life. Specifically, the severity of people's underlying heart problem is a poor predictor of their employment status, and patients' performances on treadmill tests barely correlate with their scores in detailed 'Quality of Life' questionnaires – until their cardiac condition is very poor. Thus people born with only one useful ventricle can grow up, work hard and have fun, and people who have had an apparently straightforward operation may be unemployed and sorry for themselves.

When we look beyond cardiac disability for explanations for someone's unemployment, we realize that an expectation of joining the workforce is a message fostered effortlessly in most 'normal' kids but perhaps not received by all heart children. Even now, for some their outlook is in some way provisional and it would be unsurprising if that sometimes also limited their drive. Do you ask a child 'What are you going to be when you grow up?' if you are not even certain that the child *will* grow up?

★   ★   ★

'How long have I got?' is the question that patients with cancer ask their oncologists. Will they have time to plan their funeral/

make peace with their son/write their book/bury their parents? Tell them one year and they make one plan, tell them ten years, they make another. One patient with a complicated heart repair asked the 'how long' question at her first 'adult' clinic – it was her earliest chance to enquire without her mother hearing the response. She felt that the 'twenty-year stretch ahead' gave her permission to crack on with her life. But doctors are often cagey about answering these questions. If a patient has a genuinely new heart operation today, it will be many years before prognostications are more than just an informed guess.

The last and most difficult common defect to be tackled surgically has been the Hypoplastic Left Heart Syndrome (HLHS), a problem characterized by its tiny and useless left-heart structures that fail to deliver enough forward flow to keep the babies stable after birth. When I was first in training, these newborns would arrive by ambulance looking blue and shocked. If we suspected the diagnosis, we would ask the ambulance men to wait in the canteen, take the baby to the catheter laboratory, shoot an angiogram which gave us the characteristic picture of a tiny aorta, wrap the baby up and send it back to the maternity hospital so that he or she might die with family around.

Though surgical attempts to keep such babies alive had been made previously, the first report of the first stage of what has come to be the current 'standard' three-stage plan for this lesion came out in 1980.* This initial baby surgery does not last for more than a few months of growth before the child becomes unstable again. To reach later childhood requires survival through at least two further operations. Who knows what parents of these early babies were told about the long-term outlook; my guess is that the surgeons'

---

* This came to be called the 'Norwood' operation. Like the 'Fontan' procedure, it has become an umbrella term for all the subsequent variants, each of which was aimed at improving shortcomings in the previously accepted version.

offers focused only on the very short term and parents made their decisions through the prism of knowledge that their baby would certainly die without surgery. The discourse was around 'What is the best chance of my baby being alive in one month?'

Even if every child who was operated had been kept track of from the early days (which they were not), it would be at least the year 2000 before any hospital could actually look back and do the sums to answer the question that was never asked at the time – 'Is my baby likely to reach the age of twenty?' When they did come, those calculations suggested that the early 1980s surgeons would have been correct if they had claimed that operated babies had a 20 per cent chance of surviving to the age of twenty. By the year 2000, of every five parents who had submitted their babies to surgery in the early 1980s, four had already watched their children die. Meanwhile, between 1980 and 2000, many modifications were made to each of operative stages one to three and it was clear that short- and long-term survival was improving. But even now, 'How long have I got, doc?' remains very difficult to answer for people with HLHS, especially as mechanical heart devices may be developed by the time some current patients develop the late problems that some of the early patients are beginning to experience.

★   ★   ★

Historically many youngsters were simply not expected to survive. 'Make the most of him while you've got him' was what Robert's mother was advised when he was born in 1951 (he had a single ventricle); she told him that story on this sixty-second birthday. Susan was born in the same era; her father took her boyfriend aside to warn him that she was 'not good' and 'unlikely to survive beyond the age of twenty-one'. Susan heard about that conversation on their fortieth wedding anniversary. Of course it is amusing when doctors get predictions so wrong, but doctors' credibility was at an all-time-high in the early days of the treatment of children's hearts.* Imagine being a parent constantly waiting for your child to die – pessimism must surely have an insidious effect on a child's upbringing and ambition.

So what can limit what a heart child makes of their adult life? Briefly: overprotective parenting, losing out on education, uninformed (or simply absent) careers advice, the ignorance of others as well as – just sometimes – an intelligent child's realistic appraisal of their situation. First, from home, a child may absorb bit by bit a vague sense of some restriction of their prospects. As they get older, children try to make sense of mysterious conversations between doctors and parents. Some parents' anxiety and panic gets in the way of their grasping even an upbeat message coming from medical staff and – consciously or unconsciously – a few parents even constrain children who are actually very well. Such children may have smaller dreams. At its extreme, parents can become invested in their children being 'invalids'. Some believe that this is the background to the 'learned helplessness' that leaves some survivors crippled by a minor condition.

But before we get on to the mother-blaming bandwagon, it is worth remembering what some mothers have had to deal with. Alan was a 1960s English baby – an only child with Fallot's tetralogy and a very anxious mother. When they had no surgery to offer a blue baby, it was common for doctors to caution, 'Don't let him cry.'† Youngsters with Fallot's in particular can look terrifyingly blue when upset and sometimes develop 'spells' as their circulating oxygen levels fall. Crying can progress to scary deep and rapid breathing ('air hunger'), then to a limp faint, then occasionally to

---

* They were even dragged in to advertise cigarettes: 'More doctors smoke Camels than any other cigarette.'

† 'Must wear a vest' was another one – told to Xerxes's mother. The family lived in tropical Zanzibar but childhood photos show how seriously a doctor's advice was taken.

convulsions and even death. Alan had frequent spells. He would spell after eating, spell when he woke up, spell while outside fooling around with his cousins. Twice he spelled on the toilet and fell down the hole. 'Don't let him cry' set the tone for his poor mother's parenting style; she had to carry all the responsibility for superintending her son day and night for a full five years before Alan had the chance of an operation. Little wonder that even after surgery, she remained overbearingly protective – she would not let him lock the bathroom door until he was well into his teens and banned him from sports even when he could win the races.

Cocooning can happen at school, or at work, or in the gym – often in the name of 'precaution'. Sometimes restrictions are proportionate to the problems the child has (no cross-country running is the usual example), but not always. One girl born in 1968 had her corrective operation when she was three, but obviously took her scar to school. Though perfectly well, she was constantly being controlled in what she was allowed to attempt, probably in the guise of 'sensible concern' – pulled out of the pool before completing a sponsored swim that she knew she could easily have finished. More than ten years after her corrective surgery, the careers advice she received as a teenager boiled down to: 'You have a heart problem, you need a desk job, go and train as a secretary.' Fortunately, this was a girl who was selective about the advice she took. She hit her teenage years with a vengeance, went off to town and got her ears pierced (discouraged for a heart patient)* and later trained as a nurse. Still fully fit, she likes to go to the gym where her instinctive

---

* Yes, she developed endocarditis. Before and after surgery, most patients are cautioned to avoid body piercings and tattoos because skin breaches can so easily get infected and bugs travelling in the bloodstream can settle inside their unusual hearts. Treating endocarditis takes needles, antibiotics and weeks of hospital treatment and can cause more heart damage. (That said, some people get away with piercings and tattoos.)

honesty is frequently tested – when she fills in the introductory form, should she tick a box asking about 'heart problem'? Some gyms have turned her away – one jobsworth receptionist simply said, 'You are probably better off not bothering to exercise.' Many survivors tell stories of how they can be more limited by the pre-conceptions of others than by their own physical limitations. The upshot of other people's over-reaction is the reason patients usually give for not telling employers about previous surgery.

Realistically, the childhood repairs of many congenital diseases do not confer a normal heart, and in practice, some vocations are completely barred to people who have had heart surgery, pri-marily the armed forces. That said, be impressed by the Fallot survivor with Olympic gold medals for snowboarding, the guy with a Senning operation who works as a fire-fighter and the Tunisian woman who had four successful pregnancies after a Fontan pro-cedure – few of us without scars could keep up with these people. They are truly exceptional.

When the heart cannot deliver heavy work, a decent edu-cation is a good investment. We met Patrick having a shunt for Fallot's tetralogy and learning to walk on the Manchester children's ward where he was treated. Months later he went back to his cha-otic family. Subsequently school had proved a misery and Social Services never got the measure of his household, even after his baby sister was found dead at home of malnutrition and pneumonia. He had his Fallot repair when he was thirteen; by then was getting dizzy, blue and cold. He never really returned to education after his operation and by sixteen had no qualifications and could barely read. He tried working as a hotel porter and later in a slaughter-house – though the Saturday girl could heave more than he could. At an outpatient visit after an aborted third operation, he had tried to disguise his misery from his surgeon. This man had known him ever since he had been the ward's 'little professor' and knew him to be an essentially bright lad. 'You'll kill yourself with such a strenuous job,' he told him. From a drawer, the surgeon produced a brochure; on the cover was a neatly dressed boy with an attentive teacher leaning over him – a prospectus for a residential college for disabled young people. The surgeon had been at school with the principal. He would write to him. For Patrick, this was an utterly unexpected and wonderful opportunity, both to get away from his abusive stepfather and to catch up with his education.

Catching up was tough. In a preliminary class, each student had to read a paragraph aloud – even the boy with cerebral palsy managed, though his speech was hard to understand. When it came to Patrick's turn, he bolted for the toilet. The next time he faked a nosebleed. At nineteen years of age, the humiliation of not being able to read felt overwhelming, and kind words from the teacher triggered uncharacteristic tears. When the tutor said, 'I'm afraid you will struggle to keep up,' Patrick thought his dreams were over. But a solution was found. There was a remedial class and Patrick must have been a rewarding student. Living away from home for the first time, he also had some fun, messing about with the college band ('the Cripps'). With decent qualifications, he left to train as a nurse. He was an object of fascination in the otherwise female nurses' home. Another trainee offered him a drink while he was ironing his uniform – and this was how he met his future wife. That clinic visit when a surgeon offered him an education had changed the course of Patrick's life.

Patrick worked as a health visitor until his employers panicked at his propensity to collapse with dramatic heart-rhythm troubles, sometimes while out in the community at work. The local cardiologists did their best to sort his problems, but with three young children and a dicky heart, he lost his job. Reminiscent of the man in the *Full Monty* film, he did not tell his wife, but would leave the house in the mornings and drift about terribly demoralized – until the cardiac clinic contacted his home, concerned that he was not attending appointments. His wife guessed what had happened, greeted him 'with a frying pan' and sent him back to follow up. A new round of interventions – a percutaneous pulmonary valve, an ablation, an ICD* – followed in turn. Barred from working as a nurse, he went back to university to study theology and is now the priest for a deprived inner-city parish. The last time his ICD fired, he was in a lift in an old people's home on his way to visit a dying woman. For some years, he has been the informal vicar of the local 'Grown-Up Congenital Heart' community, conducting weddings (including GUCH patient to GUCH patient) and funerals.

Some people claim that to succeed in the workplace they have to try harder than everyone else and this may well be true for adults born with heart disease. As examples to show what some determined people are capable of, we could consider some aged forty-plus who were born with only one functional pumping chamber. No operation, even now, can offer to build a normal heart from this starting point. Before the 1980s, only 'outside the heart' operations could be offered, aimed at optimizing a child's lung-blood flow so that it was not too low but not too high and so keeping the patient not too blue but not too breathless. This balance is hard to judge but, at its best, it is compatible with quite a long life – for all that it will be one branded with blueness and the tiredness that goes with it. I spoke to one man, now sixty-four, who has only ever had one childhood shunt operation. Despite his blueness and chronic fatigue, he worked conscientiously for almost thirty years, mainly doing thirty-five-hour weeks of shift-work for Post Office Telephones. Another woman, now fifty, has two scars from childhood palliative operations. To get to her office,

---

* See later. Percutaneous Pulmonary Valve Implantation: some valves can be replaced without surgery now. Ablation: another catheter-based intervention aimed at disrupting abnormal heart rhythms. ICD or Implantable Cardioverter Defibrillator: a pacemaker-related device that delivers a shock to the heart when dangerous rhythms threaten.

she needed to drive – and to set off early enough to get a car-park space; her desk was on the third floor, but there was a lift. From her early twenties to the age of thirty-six, she did not take a single day off work. In her mid thirties, she noticed that she was even more exhausted than her colleagues who had been up all night with their babies, but only went to her doctor when her ankles began to swell. (It offended her vanity that she could only get her brown shoes on when she wanted to wear a black skirt – it had not crossed her mind that her heart was playing up.) Her heart muscle was too tired for another operation to be an option and, though medicines helped, she never quite got her verve back after that time.

Gradually during the 1980s a conceptually different operation, the Fontan procedure, was offered to some. The Fontan operation 'buys' pinkness (full oxygen saturation in the body's arteries) at the price of a slightly low overall output of the heart and high pressure in the body's veins. The surgeon redirects the blue blood as it arrives back via the big veins and diverts it straight into the lung artery. From there, it flows through the lungs without the benefit of the pumping function normally performed by the right ventricle. The lungs provide the oxygen and return the red blood to the single ventricle, which then pumps it around the body. The Fontan operation has undergone many modifications and is now the 'definitive palliation' for patients born with the many varieties of single ventricle.

Wendy is now forty-two and had a Fontan operation in its very early days. When she and her mother took the coach all the way from Wales to see the important London cardiologist, Wendy was eight years old and frail, and the local doctors had nothing more to offer. This was a big outing, so Wendy was dressed in her red Ra-Ra skirt with a white trim, her red patent shoes and her white blouse with a dicky bow. From the outpatient waiting area, Wendy and her mother heard some argy-bargy, including an authoritative woman's voice, coming from the room they were heading for. It had never before crossed her mind, but her mother suddenly realized that they had come all this way to see a *woman* doctor – and that everything was going to be fine. And so it turned out. A couple of months later, Wendy was back in London for her big operation and twenty-five years after that, on a trip to the pyramids, she went to see Cairo University from where the surgeon who had carried out her Fontan had graduated.

Between those dates, Wendy gave life her all; she felt she had been given a chance on the day of the Fontan. The operation had never been 'sold' as curative nor had it given her remotely normal stamina, but from the age of eight she had a sense of needing to cram in all her goals and ambitions. From her teenage years, she had a notional 'bucket list'. From the age of fifteen, she knew she wanted to do social work to 'make a difference'. Fatigue made school a struggle, but she was single-minded. In her university years she lived at home and her family would cook when she did not have the energy; she had no student life, rarely went out and was in bed by ten. But this was all an expression of her own priorities; she felt 'fully herself', graduated with a good degree and started to work. Her first part-time job in a family centre only brought in enough money to pay for petrol – she could not possibly have managed without a car. She went on to work in youth offending, child protection and completed her social work diploma, including all the necessary placements. She worked uncompromisingly in her beloved career until clients began asking, 'Are you okay?' Assessing her for retirement on health grounds when she was thirty-nine, the doctor said he felt humbled by what she had achieved.

★   ★   ★

A staple of silly-season news is a piece about National Happiness (Denmark usually 'wins' in the happiest-country stakes). It turns out that quite a lot is known about the correlates of happiness. In surveys, 'good health' usually has the most striking connection with happiness, closely followed by 'employment' (both of these are well behind 'income' in predicting happiness). Living in a 'married or stable relationship' generally comes third. A survey of twenty- to forty-six-year-olds with the whole spectrum of repaired congenital heart disease showed that they were about as commonly married (72 per cent) as their peers. (Though the statisticians counted marriage *per se*, we all know that it is love and the company of a partner through life that promotes contentment.)

Patients look back on their youthful insecurities about building relationships as congenital heart survivors. Several spoke of hesitating to 'jump into bed' with just anyone – how would the other person react to their scar, how would they themselves cope with the questions? One woman describes feeling that 'No one would ever want me' – so when she was twenty and an offer came up, she got married rather quickly. This turned out to be a great mistake – though she did find love in the end.

Laura is in her early thirties and had two childhood operations, a Senning (see page 277) and insertion of an external tube/conduit to bypass some blockage between heart and lungs; together these add up to a far from anatomically corrected heart. As a teenager, she kept all this from her contemporaries; they were carefree and looked no further ahead than finishing their education. By contrast, Laura took nothing for granted. At eighteen, she was using her transition clinics to think through the implications of ever getting pregnant – might she make herself ill? Would it be fair to the child? At university she was extremely reticent about mentioning her heart background to her not-too-serious boyfriends. Leaving university, she had decided not to have children and prepared herself to be alone in the future, independent. Her life's simple ambition was to find a niche where she could be 'happy being happy'. She works, but is not driven by ambition or high pay – and incidentally has a lovely relationship.

Simon is perhaps more driven. His mother was already pregnant with him in 1971, when his sister died in the aftermath of a

Mustard operation for Transposition of the Great Arteries. Months later, Simon was born with the same problem. The local team helped his fearful parents obtain a second opinion in London, and Simon had the second arterial switch operation for transposition ever performed in England in 1976. Things have not gone completely smoothly since then, with reoperations and rhythm problems, but Simon feels that his sister's death confers on him a responsibility to get out and get on with life. He works hard as a psychiatric nurse, sometimes doing stints abroad for medical charities. He lists caving, bungee-jumping, skydiving and cycling among his hobbies. But while he is happy to go to Vilnius for a friend's stag weekend, there will not be one for him – he is planning not to marry. His life has turned up medical surprises to the extent that travel insurance is getting rather expensive. Now in his forties, he is very family-orientated and loves his nephews and nieces, but he does not want to take responsibility for anyone else.

16

Having a baby – what's the big deal?

amantha had surgery for an Atrioventricular Septal Defect in 1983, when she was four years old; the operation repaired the big hole where the atrial and ventricular septums join. Within a few years she was fainting, breathless and having to be carried from room to room. As a nine-year-old she listened horrified as a clinic doctor rolled a piece of paper up into a tight tube to illustrate to her parents that the way out of her left ventricle was getting smaller and smaller. (Before her second operation to relieve this obstruction, these alarming conversations triggered nightmares involving a man with a machete cutting her in half from head to chest.) In fact the surgery went well and she grew up and fell in love. During the marriage preparation course at their church, Samantha and her future husband Mark talked honestly about their desire to have children. Though no doctor had ever explicitly warned against pregnancy, her backstory had left Samantha with a dread that the obstruction might come back and she did not want to embark on motherhood unless she could expect to see her children grow up. A few years later, Samantha attended her first meeting of an 'Adult Congenital Heart' patient support group. This was the very first time she had met others in her situation and was delighted to hear their stories of motherhood. She had never considered speaking to a *heart* doctor about pregnancy and left resolving to talk to her cardiologist. Told to 'go ahead', Samantha and Mark now have two sons. The pregnancies were well monitored but went smoothly. Those boys would never have existed without that support group meeting.

Our culture is so addicted to admiring extraordinary endeavours and making celebrities of the people who achieve them that we forget that the ordinary endeavour of having a baby can be extraordinary too. More than most, women after heart operations have a lot to consider before embarking on motherhood. Elite athletes (and racehorse trainers) know that pregnancy is excellent exercise for the heart.* From very early pregnancy, the whole body gears up to its new tasks. It manufactures more blood, the heart beats a little faster and each beat – day and night – pumps out a bigger volume. By twelve weeks of pregnancy, the heart is doing 30 per cent more work than it did before. Later, the matter of lugging all the extra weight around adds to the 'training'. It is the placenta that is demanding all this extra blood flow; it services the fetus and provides all the oxygen and nutrients it needs to grow. The placenta is very greedy and can divert blood from other organs – 'low'-pertension rather than 'high'-pertension is a feature of most pregnancies, which is why pregnant women can feel wobbly when they first get up from the sofa. When it comes to the delivery room, there is another barrage of demands on the heart. The last stage of pushing a baby out is strenuous exercise and blood surges into the heart during contractions – and then most women lose over half a pint of blood after delivery. All in all, it is

* To the extent that 'Abortion Doping' was a rumoured tactic of East German athletes in the 1970s and 1980s. Allegedly, they would be artificially inseminated and then about two months later abort the unwanted fetus in time for a big event. Like much doping gossip, the stories are hard to substantiate.

easy to understand why evolution leaves pregnancy to the young and heart-fit.

From the baby's side, if blood flow to the placenta is marginal the fetus cannot prosper. If the flow is okay but the oxygen level in the mother's blood is low, the baby is also threatened. In either case, there comes a time in these precarious pregnancies when the baby's growth is so jeopardized that either miscarriage occurs or the baby is born early and small, with all the hazards that this entails. Drugs are another issue to think about; drugs that may be good for the mother may not be good for the fetus. Then there is the worry that matters to the men too – the concern that a parent's congenital heart disease is going to recur in the baby (although this turns out to be rare if the parent is the only person with congenital heart disease in the extended family). In summary, there is a lot to talk about when a woman with congenital heart disease goes to her cardiologist to think through the possibility of pregnancy: will I survive my child's childhood, will I even survive the pregnancy, will the baby be okay?

Cardiologists looking after the first wave of survivors of congenital heart surgery could not advise women with the confidence they can offer today – until the 1960s and 1970s there had never in the history of the world been pregnant women with scars on their hearts. Now some of the people who have contacted me are grandparents, and there is a whole lineage of people who would not be here but for an 'ancestor's' heart surgery.

These days a cardiologist may simply say, 'Fine, go ahead' – indeed most women who have had a repair of a straightforward problem can reasonably expect to manage. If they are taking no drugs and have a heart that can step up its output, there will probably be no problem.

But in other situations, the cardiologist may simply say, 'Whatever you do, don't get pregnant.' A heart on the brink of failing – a heart that can barely pump enough to provide for everyday demands – may never recover from a pregnancy. The increase in the volume of blood overstretches the heart muscle and, regardless of the outcome of the pregnancy, precious function may be irretrievably lost. Even worse is a circulation that cannot raise its output because of obstruction somewhere – a tight valve, a too-small artificial tube or perhaps the whole lung circuit may be restrictive, as in Eisenmenger syndrome. These dangers are not trivial; both mother and baby can die.

This is the situation in which Diana found herself. Born with 'congenitally corrected transposition'* with a Ventricular Septal Defect (VSD) and unoperated through her childhood, her lung-blood vessels became progressively damaged. Away from parental exhortations to take it easy, Diana threw herself at university life, even trying caving – setting off at dawn in a minibus full of hungover young men, climbing into cold, dark caves in Yorkshire. Dangling on a rope at the top of an underground waterfall, soaked, freezing, exhausted and unable to breathe, she met her limit (and was banned from any more expeditions by the cave-rescue team). She enjoyed sex, was really shocked when told of the danger of pregnancy and took a year to think over the advice about what to do. She was working, partying and travelling hard – she had a life worth living. But at the age of twenty-three, in the middle of her PhD and with huge ambivalence, she had a sterilization operation. She has been turning that decision over in her mind ever since. Now a highly qualified psychologist, she has noticed the repercussions of childlessness on herself and others. At first, she watched herself shut down from relationships in the aftermath of

---

* How's this for a complicated heart: the right atrium is connected to the left ventricle which is connected to the pulmonary artery. The left atrium is connected to the right ventricle which is connected to the aorta. Think this through and you notice that the blue blood eventually gets to the lungs and the red to the body. But VSDs are difficult to close in this situation and in the 1950s, nobody was offering to do it.

her sterilization, expecting to remain single, feeling she was 'damaged goods'. Then she married briefly, but her partner realized he wanted kids and they parted. With a new and much tested partner,* she looked at adoption, but was turned down on the grounds of health. They have never been one of the 'Hooray we don't have children' couples who extol the perks of childlessness. It was never a matter of choice and remains a great sadness.

Finally, a cardiologist might say, 'Well you could try,' and then come to some agreement about how to manage; each 'deal' is tailored to the woman and her particular heart. In her twenties, Chloe wanted children and the pact she made with her cardiologist was that she would spend the whole of the last three months of her pregnancy in hospital. She was a bit blue and limited but worked and managed most everyday stuff. Her heart was one of those with only marginal ability to increase its output. (She was born with Ebstein's anomaly – the right side of her heart was badly built, the muscle peculiar, the valve inefficient and a hole allowed blue blood to escape into the left (wrong) side of the heart.) She spent tedious months doing crochet in a side-ward wondering if all this precaution was a waste of time, but after her sole foray out of hospital her condition deteriorated and after that she was not even allowed out of bed. Her memory of her second pregnancy was also of terrible exhaustion.

A mother taking medicines will have another anxiety – what she needs can conflict with what the baby needs. One important example is the family of drugs that 'thin the blood' – anticoagulants. Anticoagulant treatment is recommended after some heart

---

* Diana's partner has seen her through her decline into a wheelchair needing twenty-four-hour oxygen, through the decision to be listed for a heart and double lung transplant, through the operation and through the remorseless first post-operative year – and back to work. See her wonderful book *Will I Still Be Me*?

operations; without anticoagulants, little clots can form – perhaps on the exposed metal of some valve replacements or in circulations where there are areas of sluggish flow. The two commonest anticoagulants used are warfarin – first used as a rat-poison – and heparin. Heparin is a big molecule, too big to cross the placenta or to be absorbed into the bloodstream from a dose taken by mouth; it needs to be given straight into the bloodstream, either into a vein or injected under the skin from where it can be absorbed gradually. This makes heparin an 'in-hospital' drug. By contrast, warfarin can be absorbed when taken by mouth and is manageable at home. However, it too is a tricky drug because there is a fine and rather unpredictable line between overdosing and bleeding (too much warfarin) and underdosing and clotting (too little). To wait for evidence either way is to wait too long – the consequences of bleeding or clotting can be so quickly catastrophic – so patients on warfarin are locked into having frequent blood tests to check that they are not over- or under-dosed. For many, walking that tightrope by adjusting doses in response to blood tests is a relentless preoccupation,[*] and for many patients the never-ending blood tests are the main downside of having a metal valve replacement.

Pregnancy only adds to these problems. At the best of times, pregnant women have a tendency to develop blood clots,[†] so for those with metal valves in their hearts, getting their valves bunged up with clots is a particular hazard. Erring on the side of taking a bit too much warfarin might be tempting, but that has a drawback. If a small bleed starts in the region where the baby's placenta is

---

[*] Warfarin tablets are made in nine different doses in nine different colours so that, by taking combinations of tablets, people can aim to get their total dose exactly right.

[†] Pregnancy promotes changes in clotting factors that make the blood 'hyper-coagulable'; this may be an evolutionary adaptation to minimize maternal bleeding after birth.

embedded into the wall of the mother's womb, the placenta can fall away and the pregnancy is lost. Also, warfarin can cross the placenta from the mother's to the baby's circulation; a high maternal dose will necessarily lead to a high fetal dose – and babies can bleed too. And there is another worry: when doctors started reporting the first pregnancies completed on warfarin, it emerged that the drug sometimes caused quite scary fetal malformations.*

To show how hard some people will work for a baby, meet Gemma – now an expert on all these risks. Born blue in 1979, her parents were told to expect the worst. Like Chloe, she had Ebstein's anomaly, a thin-walled, inefficient right ventricle and a hole between the two collecting chambers. She had an operation at nine years of age, another at fifteen and another at nineteen when a metal prosthesis replaced her wonky tricuspid valve. Each operation had made her a little better and the final one (with a pacemaker) had her out at work and having fun with her friends – a settled time.

She had a 'his mum knew my mum' boyfriend who came out well from an 'if we are serious, there may be no kids' conversation and they married. A few years passed and thoughts turned to pregnancy. After a raft of tests, Gemma's doctor felt that her heart was up to it, but the anticoagulation regime mandated by her metal valve could prove a problem. With Gemma's wellbeing as his priority, he recommended that she planned to continue her warfarin, with very frequent blood checks. But motherhood's protective instincts for her baby kicked in even before there *was* a baby and Gemma was swayed by the hazards that warfarin would

---

* Drugs that do this are called teratogens. Photographs of the terrible limb malformations caused by the thalidomide prescribed for morning sickness in the 1950s had horrified both doctors and parents and both were very fearful of any drug that could cross the placenta. In time, evidence emerged that warfarin was not in the same league as thalidomide as a threat, but fears of two-headed calves or babies with an eye in the middle of their foreheads are still around.

represent for the fetus. Reporting pregnant to her family doctor, she came off her warfarin and dosed herself only with aspirin, which has some anticoagulant properties.

At fourteen weeks of pregnancy, Gemma felt a pain in her shoulder. Hospital tests suggested that a clot had formed on her valve, come unstuck and landed in her lung; scans suggested the baby was okay. Gemma was persuaded back onto warfarin and everyone was happy for a couple of months – the twenty-week baby-scan looked fine and the midwives were upbeat. At work soon after, Gemma realized that she had not felt the baby move and popped in with her mother for a check-up. 'We get lots of these,' said the sonographer, quite chirpy. But with the 'camera' on her belly and the ensuing moment's silence, Gemma 'just knew'. Her fetus was dead. The sonographer was 'ever so sorry'; every-one cried. A doctor told her to stop her warfarin in anticipation of delivering a stillborn baby and sent her home with a tablet to take a couple of days later to start off the labour.

Back in hospital, her husband couldn't bear watching Gemma in pain, knowing what was ahead: a very lonely, sad labour. She did not want to look at the child at first, but after a couple of days a kindly woman came to enquire about a burial. More tears, some photographs, a blessing and a funeral followed. A post-mortem examination showed that the baby had died from bleeding into the brain – when you anticoagulate a mother you anticoagulate the fetus too. But this was not the end of the episode. Back on warfarin, Gemma continued to bleed. Three weeks later, she was still passing clots. Fed up with 'don't worry' reassurances, she and her mother headed back to hospital where she fainted in the toilet and pandemonium ensued. Resuscitation teams descended with drips, blood, plasma. She collapsed during surgery to clear out her womb. She very nearly died.

Back home Gemma resolved that she was 'not doing that again', went back on the mini-pill and thought for a while about surrogacy

or adoption. But as time passed she started trying to win round her husband, her mother and later her doctor for another try. The medical conversation was much the same the second time around and once again Gemma could not be persuaded to stay on warfarin. Aspirin and a new anticoagulant Enoxaparin (which she gave herself by injection) was the compromise: 'Your life, your body' said the doctor as he agreed the deal. Pregnant again, a regime of weekly blood tests started and progress was fine until twenty-eight weeks when a baby-scan turned up some concern about the fetus's kidneys – Gemma was huge, with a massive belly and lots of fluid in her womb. She became tired and breathless and went into hospital for bed-rest. At thirty-two weeks she was offered a test to check if the baby had a major genetic problem, but she declined – they would know soon enough. She herself got more and more short of breath, which worried the cardiologists, and an elective Caesarean section was arranged to get the baby out. The day was a Wednesday and the operating room was buzzing with doctors, but the atmosphere was joyful. Gemma remembers how they all laughed when, in the middle of the proceedings, a phone call came in from a zoo asking the obstetrician if she would do another C-section – this time on a gorilla.*
Gemma's baby came out and cried on cue, a respectable weight on the scales, had his picture taken and went off to the neonatal unit.

The next day, Gemma was still not feeling right and on the Friday she had another 'You just know . . .' scan on her heart. Her metal valve was not moving, stuck in the open position. This had been the cause of her swelling; she was going to need another operation soon. In denial she pleaded, 'Can't you just give me some medicine, I haven't got time for this,' but the cardiologist was completely intransigent, moved her from the maternity hospital to the cardiac hospital, got other operations cancelled and set her up for an emergency re-replacement of her tricuspid valve on Monday

---

* 'Would love to . . .!' was the reply.

morning. The weekend of waiting was awful, her husband shuttling between hospitals taking photos in one direction and expressed breast milk the other. The heart surgeon gave her an '80 per cent chance of no problems'.* With hormones wobbling, Gemma was left in a tangle of emotions. But she was completely surrounded by kindness. Everyone had heard the story of what she had put herself through and everyone was invested in her and the efforts she had made for her child. The obstetrician visited the cardiac hospital to check on her. As a complete surprise, the whole neonatal transport team turned up in her room with her baby in an incubator apologizing that 'they couldn't stay long'. 'Something clicked', and Gemma became the most positive person in the hospital. She made a bargain with God. 'Lets go for it. I'm fine.'

On Monday morning, she was taken straight into the operating theatre. The anaesthetist said, 'Think of something nice – perhaps your first Christmas with your baby . . .' and she was out. She woke in the early afternoon in intensive care when her obstetrician arrived with a hug saying, 'Well, I can sleep properly tonight.' She was out of bed the next day and home on Friday, ten days after her delivery and five days after her fifth open-heart operation.

Like a petite, determined motivational speaker, Gemma's advice to everyone around is 'Life is short', 'Don't over-think', 'Regret what you have done, not things you haven't done'. Her ambition is to be the oldest Ebstein – 100 years old – and get a telegram from the queen/king. My sense is that she could talk anyone into anything. Her baby is now four with no kidney problems, a Red Arrows fan. Gemma is *not* getting pregnant again but *is* expecting another baby. Her surrogate lives a few hours' drive away – and that is an extraordinary story in itself.

---

* Smart man – watch the 'framing'. If you were a new mother, would you prefer an operation with 80 per cent chance of no problems or one with 20 per cent chance of a major problem?

17

Rhythm problems and other woes: the rise of the expert patient

Stephen remembered nothing of the operation he had for Transposition of the Great Arteries (TGA) when he was ten months old. He had been sporty at school and grew up as tall as a Viking. He did a stint of travelling and at twenty-two years of age had a good job working in airport security. One day he woke with his heart racing. Completely unprimed for trouble, he drove to work, but crumpled to the floor as he entered the building. One colleague started mouth-to-mouth resuscitation and another put out a call for help on the airport's public address system. Two nurses arrived from different directions. One had been waving goodbye to her family; she was a cardiac nurse and took command. The airport defibrillator seemed ancient, but there was no alternative to trying it out and by the time the ambulance appeared, a reasonable heart rhythm had been achieved.

In the hospital, Stephen was unconscious on a ventilator when his family reached him. They were told that he was unlikely to survive the night and with twenty minutes of cardiac arrest on the airport floor, brain damage was likely if he survived. His family spent the night waiting and praying outside that ICU; every approaching footstep seemed to threaten bad news. The next morning he was still there. Arriving at his bedside, his mother whispered 'Mum's here' into his ear and he opened his eyes, suddenly distressed. She was ushered out while staff settled him, but the next time the same thing happened. A couple of days later he was out of bed apparently undamaged, though frightened about what had happened. At a specialist hospital, he had an Implantable Cardioverter Defibrillator (ICD) put in – if a similar episode recurred, it was programmed to deliver a shock promptly from a lead inside his heart. The airport administration was very reluctant to take him back and returning to work required real perseverance, but he won his battle and on his refresher module he met his future wife.

'Sudden cardiac death' may be the first and last manifestation of a heart rhythm disturbance. Coming out of the blue in young people on the sports field, it hits headlines. When it happens to people who had put their congenital heart disease behind them, the emotional shock for families is awful. Stephen had a 'near miss'. By their very nature, unexpected and sinister heart rhythm changes ('arrhythmias') are difficult to research, but if a patient has clues suggesting that they are at risk, technology or drugs can sometimes help.

We all take our hearts for granted – I can go for days and days without 'remembering' that I have a heart myself. If I am not doing hard exercise, it can take an occasional extra, walloping beat to bring to mind that there is something crucial in there. We all get random 'flip-flops' in our chests and have learned not to be alarmed; even a whole string of odd beats do not usually amount to anything. Not all changes in heart rhythms cause these 'palpitations' and not all queer heartbeats are ominous. However, people with congenital heart disease often tune into their 'palpitations' and – even if these are completely benign – they may serve to remind them that they have a heart, and that their heart might not be completely reliable.

The medical specialism that deals with heart rhythms is called electrophysiology; its main diagnostic tool is the electrocardiogram (ECG). The ECG is recorded from electrodes stuck onto the skin; they detect electrical impulses rippling away from the different regions of the heart as each beat plays out in an orderly way. The beat normally starts at the top of the right atrium and propagates to and through the muscle of the ventricles. Most doctors will be able to recognize whether or not an ECG is dangerously abnormal, but it takes a specialist with a certain nerdy preoccupation with details of the orders of blips, the heights and widths of waves and the intervals between them to come to a detailed diagnosis of where in the heart the origin of an electrical problem lies.

Another difficulty in the diagnosis of arrhythmias is that they are often intermittent. A patient may have recurring complaints of breathlessness or chest pain or feeling faint or tired because of a change in her heart rhythm, but sod's law dictates that her heart will not be misbehaving while she is actually being examined in the clinic. This means that, unless someone at least considers an arrhythmia as an underlying cause, her symptoms may be completely dismissed. Like an aeroplane's 'black box', the ECG must somehow be recorded continually during everyday life if understanding of an incident is not just to be guesswork. The technology to record a 'twenty-four-hour ECG' first became available in the 1960s, when itchy stickers were put on a child's chest and their ECGs recorded on huge reel-to-reel tape machines hung around their necks as they went to school. Equipment has improved enormously and now smartphones can save the data, upload it to a computer and transmit it to a doctor or technician; some applications can even give the patient a voice message to warn them that there is mischief going on.

Abnormal rhythms can be slow or fast, regular or irregular, intermittent or constant, terrifying or benign. They may be inherent to the problem someone was born with or can originate in a surgical scar or in the wall of a heart chamber as it gradually stretches. The Mustard and Senning operations for TGA and the early versions of the Fontan operation all leave long lines of stitches in the heart's collecting chambers and few of these patients are in completely reliable normal rhythms ten years after surgery. Patients after surgery for Fallot's tetralogy all have scars where ventricular muscle has been cut or chopped away and arrhythmias – some nasty – originating in the ventricles become a major worry over time.

Unfortunately, for survivors of congenital heart surgery, getting to a heart-rhythm diagnosis is often a real difficulty. Neither the patient nor their usual doctor may even consider a rhythm problem as a possible cause of symptoms of 'commonplace' fatigue. Cardiologists without particular experience of congenital heart disease may not consider it. Even 'off the shelf' electrophysiologists may think they know what is going on, but may actually be completely out of their depth – the ECGs of congenital heart patients are almost all abnormal, even in the absence of rhythm problems. The benefit of being cared for by someone likely to recognize rhythm problems promptly is one of the best reasons for encouraging patients to stay in specialist follow-up – when people are well, it may seem tempting to drift away, but there is a lot of ignorance out there.

For example, after a childhood repair a bright young woman was transitioned 'up' to an adult cardiology clinic. In her late twenties she developed bouts of chest pain. Because chest pain in a general heart clinic usually corresponds to poor flow down the heart's own arteries, the team there did some coronary angiograms to look at her blood vessels. Unsurprisingly in a young woman, these showed no furring of the arteries – so the problem was 'in her head' and she was told, 'Have a baby, that will sort your hormones out.' Overriding this kind of 'authority' to reach a proper adult congenital heart specialist took a lot of persistence – but outrage is a great motivator.

Some experienced patients develop well-honed 'bullshit detectors'. The first clue that a doctor is out of their depth is often his need to impress the patient with his credentials. A second occasionally comes as a giveaway phrase that confirms their ignorance. An electrophysiologist keen to pick up a new patient asked one man who wanted help with his palpitations after a childhood repair, 'What side of the heart is that A-V canal of yours located in?'* The patient knew enough to keep well away from that man, but finding your way to real expertise is genuinely difficult if you are not yourself part of the medical community. Knowing you are unwell, and being patronized by a doctor who you know to be in the wrong is a very frightening position for a patient to be in. It's best never to lose touch with expertise.

Barry would agree. He spent his seventh birthday and recently his sixtieth in 'his' hospital; he had a Fallot repair in the early 1960s and has never lost contact with the unit. The original operation gave him a life, but the team have gone on 'saving' him every decade since – with improving technology. Barry's first post-operative problems were blackouts in his twenties. After coming-to while convulsing on his bed after playing badminton, he visited his family doctor. She noticed a very slow heart rate and told him to take it easy. Q. 'For how long?' A. 'For the rest of your life.' So Barry got in touch with his specialist hospital and they sorted him out with his first pacemaker. It delivered 70 impulses every minute to 'fire' his ventricular muscle continually, day and night. This was enough to stop the fainting episodes but, because he could not increase his heart rate above those 70 beats per minute, his badminton performance was dismal – and so Barry started a lifetime of being a 'guinea pig' for new technologies. A technician came to

---

* Jargon can be a self-serving language for an 'in-group', but it also clarifies who is in the 'out-group'. 'A-V canal' is shorthand for a complex hole, right in the middle of the heart.

the badminton club and monitored his pulse rate, eventually fixing him up with a pacemaker system that allowed Barry to 'dial up' his own heart rate from the outside – 70 beats per minute 'baseline' and 120 per minute for 'activity' (helpful for badminton and bedroom). Later, pacing systems were developed with the intelligence to automatically raise the pacing rate to match the body's demand on the heart; these are commonplace now. Subsequently Barry was troubled by abnormal rhythms originating in his atria, but the technology to zap the source(s) using radiofrequency waves or lasers arrived in time to help; this is a procedure called ablation. Barry is currently on his seventh pacemaker system – 'top-of-the-range' and able to deliver a shock in response to a deadly rhythm, as well as drive his heart when it is going too slowly. The subjective sensation of these devices firing is weirdly indescribable – if it occurs before you have actually lost consciousness. The feelings are muddled because the giddiness of the rhythm that triggered the shock and the shock itself merge together as the person picks themselves up off the floor and tries to process what has happened: one man said, 'It's like the inside of your chest being kicked by a horse.'

All this sounds as though well-looked-after patients with technological solutions to their arrhythmias are indestructible. The 'patient's guardian angel' is the advertising patter used by companies who sell implantable defibrillators to doctors – and doctors talk to their patients in similar terms. But this is to sugar-coat the experience of actually living with this kind of technology. Patients tell us to remember the proverb about 'walking a mile in my shoes'. Would your life-view change if you had a shock while having sex, or while you were driving, or when you were out with your children? Would you become secretive about shocks to spare your spouse's worry? Would you listen to your heart in the dead of night? People with ICDs have made a pro-life choice, but these patients live between a rock and a very hard place.

Psychological issues aside, you have to boggle at the technological advances in revamping the heart's electrics since the first start-ups emerged in the garages of Minneapolis in the 1950s. These out-fits have become huge multinational companies with eye-watering turnovers. The pulse-generator 'boxes' (that fire each pacemaker beat) have shrunk from being the size of a brick carried around an unfortunate child's neck to devices the size of an Oreo cookie that are usually implanted under the skin of the chest wall, just below the collar bone. The batteries hermetically sealed inside these units last much longer (years rather than months). The pacing wires that are threaded through a vein to deliver the electrical impulse from the pulse generator to the heart do not fracture or need fiddling with as often as they did in the old days. But even now, having metalwork in one's body is not problem-free. All veterans who have been paced for years have had trouble with wires (getting them in and getting them out) or pacemaker batteries poking through their skin and 'falling out' of their pockets – and some patients complain that siting a battery at just the wrong place on their shoulders cramps their rifle-shooting!* For some who are preoccupied by the bulges and scars over their hardware, the newest gee-whizz device may be their future. 'Leadless' pacemakers are plopped straight into the cavity of the right ventricle; on X-ray they look like a bullet in the heart. They are deployed through a vein in the leg – and may later need to be fished out the same way. Once nicely placed, these units can take over the pacing of the heart's ventricles; no scar, no lead and – everyone hopes – no bother.

Still, controlling some rhythms with drugs should be less oner-ous. Over the decades, many drugs have come on the market and, if a patient is prepared to take tablets every day, many do keep certain troubles at bay. Almost all have side effects, so it is tempting

---

* Michael, who had a Senning operation for TGA, would say that, if you choose your sport well, a pacemaker is no bar to high achievement. He has an Olympic medal to prove it (see plates).

to keep the doses as low as possible while still controlling the problem. This does mean that abnormal rhythms can break through
and patients may arrive in casualty departments with their hearts
racing, sometimes feeling mortally ill – and there may be no real
expertise at hand. This is when it is worthwhile for a patient to
carry a 'care plan' so that their specialist cardiologist can advise
the local personnel about what best to do – which drugs might
work or if an electrical shock would be the best treatment choice.
Unfortunately several patients told me stories about how these
ostensibly worthwhile documents were completely ignored. One
man teetering on the verge of unconsciousness due to his fast heart
rate saw a cluster of junior doctors at the end of his bed, looking
at textbooks to decide what to do with him. 'Just don't give me
verapamil – I'll arrest,' he said. They did – and he did.*

   But my favourite 'expert patient' story is Roy's. Roy (a Fallot
survivor), his wife and another couple were tourists in Prague,
then the capital of Czechoslovakia. On a metro platform, he began
to feel dizzy and realized – not for the first time – that his heart
rhythm was misbehaving. Strangers helped the little group to call an
ambulance and a barely conscious Roy found himself in a foreign
hospital, on a gurney with a nervous-looking doctor looming over
him. At the best of times, rhythm problems in people with scars
on their chests make casualty staff apprehensive, and the language
barrier meant that little could be learned from the patient. 'Shock'
was perhaps the limit of this man's English and down came the
paddles on Roy's bare chest and the button pressed. The pain was
beyond terrible, but he did not blaspheme. As he composed himself
after the shock, it quickly became clear that the attempt at 'cardio-
version' had not worked. Before the paddles came down again, Roy
leaned forward and turned up the voltage dial on the defibrillator,
before sinking back on the stretcher, resigned to another onslaught.

---

* He survived – and told me about it.

This time his heart reverted and Roy and the Czech doctor silently sized up the situation. Who was the expert? The patient, as *Father* Roy, worked as a hospital chaplain. In the course of his working day he had often held patients' hands while hospital teams pumped on their chests to try to resuscitate them from cardiac arrests. Often he had been told to stand back for the moment that a shock was delivered. The dial was familiar. He knew about voltage.

★ ★ ★

Unfortunately changes in the heart's rhythm are not the only snags that adults with congenital heart disease can experience. Late complications relating to defects in their hearts that were not fixed at their original operations can catch up with them many years later. However unwelcome, some troubles can be recognized in advance and faced squarely, but it is the complications that come out of the blue that rock a person's sense of control of their life.

In 1973 when Guy was born, there seemed no way to improve his complicated 'plumbing'. Until he was eight, he had been so blue and his stamina was so limited that his father had needed to carry him on his shoulders to get about. A big operation at a faraway hospital when he was nine put him on a BMX bike, then a skateboard as he rushed to make up for lost time. As a twenty-year-old art student in London, he had needed a second operation to replace a tube that had been part of his first surgery, but he got through that. After graduating he landed a hugely prestigious residency at an artist's institute in Amsterdam and, like any young man given such an opportunity, he embraced the excessive way of working of the young artist. The massive structures he made for his solo show claimed all his energy, and only afterwards did he realize that he was unmistakably ill. He coughed up some blood. He felt as if someone was sitting on his chest. His heart was pumping hard. He became disorientated. He was living alone in a foreign country before the days of mobile phones. After two days, he managed to stagger down to the street where passers-by passed by as he stumbled around erratically. A friend found him sitting on the pavement and got him to hospital, where the Dutch doctors asked, 'Is your heart usually twice the normal size?'

Over the following months every hope he had for his future seemed to disintegrate. He spent a long time in hospital; at one stage there was talk of a heart transplant. When he was eventually able to leave the ward, he had to go back to live with his parents. Instead of taking up an exciting job offer in Amsterdam, he had to apply for Incapacity Benefit. Worse, the benefits assessor who visited him at home anticipated that he would never work again and signed him on 'for life'. Guy felt that so many people – parents, surgeons and artists – had given him every possible chance and now, at the age of twenty-four, his life seemed behind him. The grief was brutal.

It took about a year of changing drug regimes to bring the infection and heart failure under control and Guy crawled back to a semblance of health. He took up an offer to visit Japan, where one of his pieces was being exhibited, and later lived there for a couple of years and married. When his cardiologist suggested that a mitral valve replacement would be a good investment for his future, his heart sank and he seriously considered declining surgery. It was concern for his young child that his wife used as her plea to clinch the decision to go ahead. Surfing the uncertainty of his future has been emblematic of Guy's whole life; at no stage since his childhood could a doctor give a confident answer to the question 'How long have I got?' In his twenties Guy was close to thinking about his own funeral; now he has two jobs and two children, friends are beginning to experience health troubles and, in his forties, he says he is 'too old to die young'.

These days the commonest operation for congenital heart disease in adult life is the replacement of pulmonary valves. Valves 'work' by closing; they maintain the circulation as a one-way system.

If a valve leaks, blood sloshes backwards and overloads the chamber it has just come out from. If a pulmonary valve is leaking, at each beat the right ventricle needs to push out all the blood that has already headed out for the lungs but slopped 'backwards', as well as the blood arriving 'forwards' from the right atrium. Amazingly, it can manage to do this without complaint for many years, but a tipping point is eventually reached. So-called 'right-heart failure' takes you down the way that Hemingway says you go bankrupt – 'gradually then suddenly'. The 'gradual' loss of fitness is often so slow that the person denies it – just like the rest of us 'fail to notice' how we gain weight in middle age. The 'sudden' crisis in right-heart failure manifests with gross swelling and exhaustion. This situation is a real misery that is hard to climb back out of, even if a new valve is put in. However, if the person is attending clinics for occasional check-ups, their cardiologist will be tracking how well their right ventricle is performing. If it is gradually failing, they may raise the issue of planning for a valve replacement at a time when the patient does not think of himself as having many symptoms.

Surgery in adult life aimed at revising shortcomings in the original repairs now represents 20 per cent of all the congenital heart operations in the UK. These are increasingly done before the patient is very symptomatic. Suggesting an operation as an invest-ment for an adult's future is a very different conversation from the one that confronted that same person's parents decades earlier when an operation was the only way their child would have any future at all. The risk-versus-benefit debate for someone who themselves has children, a job and a mortgage has to be very persuasive; the chances of dying and the time off work have to be balanced against the life-prospects without further surgery. Submitting to another big operation is especially tough for people who have grim mem-ories of previous hospital stays, often many years previously and tangled up with childhood fears. Given the choice, some are fearful and wait; others just want the operation behind them. Some old

hands simply sigh and pack their bags: 'I like to inspect the operating room,' said one.

Paul was one of these veterans; he had had three operations
by the age of seventeen. The most recent had been to replace a
conduit – an outside-the-heart tube that had been needed as part
of his main repair. Now the pictures showed that the valve in his
conduit was leaking and his lung arteries might be better with a
bit of cosmetic surgery. Even simply cutting through his sternum
for a fourth time carried some risk and, realistically, rehabilitation
after the operation would mean several months off work – but
surgery would be a good long-term investment. Paul's heart sank
and he asked for a second opinion at another hospital, which was
organized a little grudgingly. This was 2005, when an alternative
to open-heart surgery was newly achievable – a Percutaneous
Pulmonary Valve Implantation (PPVI). 'Percutaneous' implies that
this whole procedure is done in an X-ray department by a cardiologist rather than in an operating room by a surgeon. They approach
the heart from the vein at the top of the leg, take some pictures and
proceed to blow up a balloon to stretch any narrow vessels (Paul's
pulmonary arteries). If necessary, metal stents (expandable mesh
tubes) can be positioned to prop open the narrow vessels. Stents
are introduced by crimping them tightly over the deflated balloon
as it goes into the leg vein and balloon and stent are nudged up
together to the narrow area of the lung artery; when the balloon
is inflated, the stent expands and stays open after the balloon is
deflated and withdrawn.

Stents had been used in various parts of the circulation since
the late 1980s but the next step was to design a 'foldable' valve that
could be packed over a deflated balloon, wiggled into position
then unfolded to lodge inside a stent. At the time Paul needed
help, the valve procedure was still 'work-in-progress' and all the
research paperwork took time. The process of getting Paul's formal agreement to an experimental procedure kept his feet on the

ground; the operator told him explicitly about previous mishaps and about what he had learned from each of them – Paul had to hear the story of what had happened when one conduit had split and bled and how the situation had been retrieved. Also, because the valves were new, nobody could know how long they would last. But Paul went ahead and had PPVI number 110. He quickly felt much better for it. His stay in hospital was short, he had no scar and was soon cycling to work – and ten years later is happy with the decision he made.

'Intelligent' defibrillators and valve replacements performed without surgery – such technologies were undreamed of at the beginning of congenital heart treatment. Even now, many doctors have no idea of their existence. For the right patients they may add many years to their lives, but in practice they are not available to everyone who could benefit. This is not primarily an issue of cost (though the costs are whopping) but a matter of putting the right patients in front of the right doctors. Half of the patients who died many years after a Fallot repair performed in my own hospital were not under specialist follow-up at the time they died. People easily drifted out of follow-up before adult services were consolidated in the 1980s, and many have still not found their way back. Others feel well and don't turn up to appointments; we can only hope that they don't suddenly become 'bankrupt'.

I have heard many stories of how unsafe it has been for patients to be looked after by doctors who do not know the territory of adult congenital heart disease. For example, Rita had had an early 1950s operation in Boston for pulmonary stenosis* and had a scar to show for it. Previously thin and breathless, she was transformed by the surgery and would 'twist and twist again' as a teenager.

---

* A blocked pulmonary valve. In the 1950s this needed surgery, these days a balloon mounted on a cardiac catheter is passed across the valve and blown up – job (usually) done!

By the age of thirty she was chasing around after her three boys and working a thirty-hour week, but she really was terribly tired. A local cardiologist diagnosed 'housewife syndrome' ('read tired and bored'). When she eventually reached someone who at least recognized that the pulmonary stenosis had recurred – or perhaps had never been properly relieved – she came to re-operation. The orifice of her pulmonary valve through which the whole output of her right heart had to flow was the size of a pencil lead instead of being the width of a thumb. All this time, she must have had a very noisy murmur and the signs of right-heart failure must have been perfectly evident, but very few doctors would ever have seen this combination of features in a young woman who 'should' be well. Reaching competent doctors is not only crucial for the patient – without that operation, three little boys would have suddenly and inexplicably lost their mother.

In 2010, estimates suggest that around 500,000 adults in the USA and over 80,000 adults in the UK are living with 'complex' or 'moderate' congenital heart disease needing lifelong surveillance. Currently in the USA, about 9,000 young people every year should pass through the metaphorical gates between their children's and adult hospitals, 1,600 in the UK. Over a decade, this corresponds to an extra 90,000 people in the USA and 16,000 in the UK who will need help from specialists who are alert to the great variety of problems that adults with congenital heart conditions and surgery experience. The pressure of patient numbers means the clinics are often busy and the throughput of transient trainee doctors makes many 'old timers' regret that the days of seeing 'their own' cardiologist have largely gone. In many units the glue that holds the service together is the liaison nurse who is prepared to spend time on the telephone and who can hustle if necessary on a patient's behalf.

Researching this chapter, I have heard many patients' stories that reflect badly on doctors as a class of people – arrogant, patronizing and above all ignorant. It set me wondering how embarrassed

I should be. Not to excuse but to explain; adults with congenital heart disease are outnumbered twenty-five to one by people with coronary artery disease or diabetes.* A patient – child or adult – is likely to be the only one with congenital heart disease on the list of their primary-care doctor. Congenital heart disease is still barely mentioned at medical school. Most problematic is that a patient's main concern is often unaccustomed fatigue – a complaint common to so many mental, physical and lifestyle causes. In consequence of all of this, many patients can take many years and several doctors before they reach someone who recognizes the nature of their problem.

Along the way, many of these patients had been told that they were faking being sick when actually for many years they had been faking being well. A recurrent grievance is that we doctors don't know what we don't know. In our defence, I would say that we are not the only ones.† It seems a near-universal human failing and the source of most disastrous misjudgements in the worlds of war and finance as well as in medicine. The best protection a doctor can cultivate is a curiosity about every patient – here the giveaway clue is the scar of congenital heart surgery. If they notice the scar, if they have enough humility and if they carry a wide circle of competent colleagues on their phone's speed-dial, all should be well. If their patient has congenital heart disease and is not regularly seen in a specialist clinic, it seems to me indefensible not to refer them.

---

* One survivor of early major surgery was called to her family doctor for routine blood tests . . . Her cholesterol levels were fine . . . 'You'll have no problems with your heart, then,' said her doctor.

† Donald Rumsfeld: '. . . as we know, there are known knowns; there are things we know we know. We also know there are known unknowns; that is to say we know there are some things we do not know. But there are also unknown unknowns – the ones we don't know we don't know. And if one looks throughout the history of our country and other free countries, it is the latter category that tend to be the difficult ones.'

The best way a patient can help himself is to remain on the books of an experienced centre – and get in touch with the 'mother ship' if he is concerned. Knowing something about their own condition is a great help too; if remembering the details is too difficult, demand and carry a copy of a letter describing it all. Find and join a Facebook group, an internet bulletin board or a support group – you are not as alone as you think. Ask other patients for advice and courage – you are almost certainly not the first person to experience your particular problem.

18

'Death alone is certain, the time of death is uncertain'

The inside of Christine's heart was repairable, but her lung-blood supply was too weird. Instead of an artery coming directly from her heart, small vessels meandered from her aorta to supply different parts of her lung; none was very big and all were prone to silting up, so she was blue and precarious. In the late 1980s when she was five, her mother was told for the first time: 'You won't have her for long.'

While she was at primary school, two attempts were made to streamline her lung-blood supply without dealing with the inside of her heart; they helped for a while. Incongruously, at secondary school, someone carried her bag between lessons; this was a time of fairly minimal survival. But Christine delivered good exam results and went to university to study French. By the time she was eighteen, she needed a wheelchair and someone to push it. As a disabled student she received some financial and practical help, but by her second year she could not leave even her room if the lift broke down, and retreated home to her mother, defeated.

Her stamina got worse and worse. While visiting a friend, she had an episode of coughing up blood – horrible, thick, red blood. It transpired that a fungus ball was lurking in one lung; it must have started as a small airborne spore that grew gradually in the low-oxygen environment of her unhealthy lung and eventually eroded the surrounding blood vessels. She was admitted to intensive care and her mother was summoned and told for a second time: 'She hasn't got long.' But the bleeding did stop and Christine left hospital to get on with her life – and with her relationship with her loyal boyfriend.

Wayne is 6 feet 4 inches tall; Christine is tiny – she often has to wear children's clothes. She describes Wayne as geeky, loyal and patient. Wayne describes Christine as 'a mini version of Mr T in *The A-Team*,* a real softy, but with a mean streak. She gives me a look that's as dangerous as a punch! She is brave, but I can't say that to her face because she doesn't like pity – she would probably respond like the Incredible Hulk!' This gives us a flavour of how the two of them have dealt with what happened next.

When Christine was twenty-four, the massive coughing drama happened again – blood dribbling down her chin. Day and night, the coughing would not stop; hospital nurses watched helpless and in tears. In a 'make or break' gesture a young doctor gave her some sedation and the bleeding gradually subsided, though she had a stroke in the aftermath. She found the stroke terrifying – being *compos mentis* while her body wouldn't work and her speech was limited to grunting 'yes' or 'no'.

She recovered, but around this time her medical consultant broached the question of whether Christine would want to be

---

* For those who don't know, Mr T is black, weighs 255 pounds, wears bling around his torso and has a heart of gold. He cultivates a mean look and his initials are B.A. for Bad Attitude. Christine is white, and has never in her life weighed more than 84 pounds, but she certainly has 'attitude'.

resuscitated if she had another massive bleed. Obviously she was in a very bad situation, but it was also clear that it had the potential to become even worse. If she collapsed and someone put a tube down her throat to allow a machine to take over her breathing, she might be stuck in hospital on a ventilator with no exit strategy. So Christine had level-headed discussions with her mother, her sister and Wayne. Long-term hospitalization seemed a truly terrible prospect, so she signed some paperwork stating that she did not ever want to be 'saved' in this way – a 'DNR'* order.

She did seem to be approaching the end-stage of her heart condition, but the 'mini Mr T' still had a bucket list. The first job was to organize the wedding. Her mother bought the dress and Christine and Wayne married when she was twenty-five. As she had promised herself, Christine walked down the aisle – though she took her vows in a wheelchair, gulping on oxygen. Wayne took *her* surname. She threw up with exhaustion during the photos but got through the day, living on adrenaline. She would not be talked down to. If someone said, 'Aren't you brave,' she would respond, 'No, why?', while, 'Aren't you lucky,' would elicit the reply, 'No; are disabled people not meant to get married?' That said, the day was a test of her endurance. She enjoyed her first anniversary party much more – boogying in her wheelchair.

Life is 'brilliant' now that Christine and Wayne live together in an adapted flat. Her new electric wheelchair has been a real boon and worth all the assessments and 'driving tests' she needed to merit it. They have a converted car – their 'pope-mobile' – and try to get out every day. Another bucket-list item arrived in the form of Cindy, a rescue dog; she gets walks on the beach. Wayne does the cooking and housework. They are jokey and sociable, watch television, play computer games, use Facebook.

---

* DNR: 'Do not resuscitate' or 'no code'.

Christine is crafty – knitting or making cards or jewellery or mosaics. She is a bad sleeper; in one position her back hurts, in another she can't breathe. When she dreams, there is no wheel-chair; she walks, dances and even runs – something her waking body has not done for twenty years. She is on oxygen day and night. A palliative care nurse knows her well and will see her through, though Christine thinks her death 'won't be quick' and 'might be horrible'. But morale is really good; her will is written and her funeral paid for. Wayne says he will get a parrot when she dies. Still on the bucket list is reaching her thirtieth birthday. Respect to both of them!

★   ★   ★

I find it very hard to strike the right note for a chapter about death. Magazine articles about the deaths of young people usually headline with the 'tragedy' – and then try to engineer a 'feel-good' piece by spinning the positive side of the loss: the fortitude, the silver linings that can always be found. These accounts seem to me to be both true and yet fundamentally fake. I should perhaps declare my own 'dual nationality' here. As a doctor and trained in paediatric cardiology and surgery, I had seen children die many times – on the operating table, in intensive care, suddenly and unexpectedly or quietly in their parents' arms. So by the time my own child died at the age of five, I already knew that this happened to beautiful children and that beautiful families grieved. I had also witnessed how doctors and nurses are cast down by a child's death – before they need to pick themselves up again and go about their work. They may not remember every name, but each death does leave a mark. Then when death comes to your own child, you get another long, hard look at it.

It seems too difficult for me to write neatly about death, so I have cheated (or retreated) into its paradoxes – propositions that seem to be true and false at the same time.

'It would be easier and cheaper to go and make another baby.'

This quote comes from the 1950s. It conveys the gut reaction of many conservative doctors to the proposition that surgeons might cut into babies in the apparently vain hope of curing their hearts. But, even today, its lurking sentiment is not obsolete. Though the phrasing is hopefully less crass, a similar attitude sometimes surfaces when scans show pregnant women that their children will have complex and potentially lethal heart problems.

In truth, the persistence of the first surgeons who operated on children's hearts against the hostility of this 1950s attitude is what kicked off the whole raft of astonishing advances that we take for granted today. The minds of the early teams were not only on the children in front of them, but also on future children with the same problem. Looking back, the entire endeavour can seem heroic, carried out entirely for the greater good. However, it was also true that some surgeons' motivations included promoting their personal careers and status. US culture in particular rewarded clinicians for adopting bold new strategies; fame and financial gain were there for the taking. The competitive and ambitious atmosphere made for many conflicts of interest and some less-than-exemplary behaviour. It was like an environment where people could build houses without needing planning permission or building regulations. There was – and remains – no FDA* for the surgeon; a surgeon could wake up in the morning and try a brand-new operation with legal impunity.

There were some mythically gigantic egos around in the early days. 'Medical experimentalism' was essentially an extension of 'medical practice' and doctors tacitly expected their patients to

---

* FDA: the Food and Drug Administration, the enormously powerful US federal agency that regulates the arrival on the market of new drugs, vaccines, medical devices – but not new operations.

make sacrifices for the sake of medical progress. Doctors' author-
itarianism was standard and – mostly – patients just fell in line.
Surgeons did not always tell the truth to patients, parents or each
other; subtle coercion was commonplace. They publicized their
successes and hid their failures.

But it was also very tough for them. Doing something new
involved a risk to their reputations if it went wrong. Of course,
history only records the names of the victors; surgeons who failed
or did not join the chase disappear from the record. All surgeons
negotiating a 'learning curve' have to deal with the deaths of their
patients. When anyone tried to stop them operating, 'you had to
be absolutely convinced internally that you were right and that
everybody else was wrong'. Some were diabolical to their staff
yet popular with families, others the completely the reverse. But
if accounts of operations were ever published, the names of the
people who had been 'under the knife' were redacted. There has
never been the slightest acknowledgment of the debt that medicine
owes to pioneering patients.

New interventions are still being conceived, but since the
1950s when congenital heart treatment started, doctors' pater-
nalism has been gradually constrained. In response to the sadistic
'experiments' undertaken by doctors in Nazi Germany, proposals
for medical research are now scrutinized by people outside the
investigating team. In response to doctors 'failing to comply with
hospital polices regarding informed consent', doctors have been
deprived of their licence to practise.* In many other ways, medicine is more regulated now. In the 1940s, when Helen Taussig was
writing her groundbreaking book on congenital heart disease, she
would ask parents for the opportunity to look at a child's heart,

---

* Failing to comply with hospital consent procedures was how Dr Norwood
(who initially persisted in treating Hypoplastic Left Heart Syndrome) ended
his career in 2006.

even in advance of their deaths, but this discipline of transparency lapsed. Later, if an autopsy followed an operation, surgeons would surreptitiously keep back the heart when the rest of a child's body was returned for burial; they learned a lot about their surgery from these 'specimens'. In the UK, it took a change in the law to oblige teams to seek a parent's consent if they want to retain a child's heart for future learning and research.*

But more than rules, it is attitudes that change the dynamics of medicine. Somewhere behind 'Go and make another baby' and also behind 'We might as well operate, he is going to die anyway' is the sense that the patient is 'only' a baby – somehow dispensable in the scheme of things. He is a statistic, even a commodity. Try telling that to the parents of a newborn with Hypoplastic Left Heart Syndrome (HLHS). If this diagnosis comes as a surprise after birth, his parents have only a couple of hours in which to contemplate the future of their child – and of their whole family; after that, the baby will begin to decline without treatment. Looked at rationally, the human costs of embarking on surgery seem prohibitive. Parents risk sacrificing their family structure; husbands and wives often separate under the pressure and brothers and sisters are marginalized, sometimes for months at a time. Stress levels, particularly for mothers, are excessive and enduring. Parents with no support from extended families are at real risk of 'failure to cope'. Even if

---

* The 'Alder Hey scandal' broke in the UK when over 2,000 pots of children's hearts and other organs were found in the hospital's pathology department. In fact 'libraries' of abnormal hearts of dead children had for years been kept in many hospitals on both sides of the Atlantic and were actively used for research and teaching. They had significantly helped surgeons' understanding of the problems they had to fix. However their retention had been an example of doctors taking for granted that the 'rights' of medical progress necessarily trumped the 'rights' of parents to bury their children's bodies complete. In the UK, the law was clarified in 2004 but for a while the scandal impacted organ donation rates for transplantation and autopsy rates after cardiac surgical deaths.

things go well, some teenagers struggling with their Hypoplastic Left Heart repairs reproach their parents for not allowing them to die.* The financial cost of 'stage 1' surgery is also eye-watering – currently averaging \$323,045† – and there are two more major operations, countless future hospital visits, tests and an almost certain loss of parental income to take into account. Embarking on this path is far beyond the financial means of most families outside of an adequately insured or publicly funded healthcare system. A country does not have to be very poor before money influences its whole society's attitude to babies with serious congenital defects; its public can see reason in letting babies die. (From the perspective of our privilege, we call this 'fatalism', but some cultures may be more resilient than we are in the face of death.) These are the facts for babies with HLHS and their families *in general*.

But *particular* parents only make decisions for their *own* baby and need to take account of nobody other than their other children, to whom they also owe parental protection. Surgery is the baby's only chance of still being alive in one month; 'comfort care' is the name given to the alternative. This involves tending to the baby and surrounding him with love until he dies. In making the decision of whether or not to embark on a series of operations and an uncertain future, facts, emotions, cultural and religious pressures all collide differently in different families. In the short term, 'comfort care' is probably the tougher option for parents to choose. To watch their precious child die in their arms when there is an alternative, they need to be like those early surgeons who were convinced internally that the decision was right. It is a delicate area to research, but parents with more extended education are marginally more likely to opt for 'comfort care'; this includes people with a medical background. In contrast, and for

---

* Some teenagers without these problems do that too.
† And some 3 per cent cost over \$1 million, just for 'stage 1' of three stages.

all sorts of reasons, most families do not hesitate to choose – even demand – an operation.

In England, in more than half of pregnancies affected, HLHS is recognized before birth and parents have a little more time to think. Scans can pick up the characteristic picture at around twenty weeks' gestation, by which time all these babies are very much wanted.* Some parents know immediately what they will do; others appreciate help with their choice. 'Decision support' can take many forms; social media can put parents in touch with others who have been in the same situation. In some jurisdictions where termination of pregnancy for fetal abnormality is available, over 60 per cent of parents given the diagnosis of HLHS in their unborn child terminate the pregnancy. There are even support groups that bear witness to the pain of parents who have ended a wanted pregnancy. It is clear that termination of pregnancy is not an 'easy' option, but it is definitely even harder to stand back and decline surgery after the baby is born.

I'm guessing that the guy who said, 'It would be easier and cheaper to go and make another baby' had never himself had a child with congenital heart disease. I'm guessing too that surgeons who steamrollered naive parents into novel operations, including the early Hypoplastic Left Heart operations, might have negotiated differently with a medical colleague who had an affected baby. To me, the paradox is how these boorish types who tell people what to do can be both right and so profoundly wrong at the same time.

---

* This is worth saying because in much of Europe over 25 per cent of all pregnancies are electively terminated, almost all in the early weeks; we might say that these pregnancies were unwanted. By inference, fetuses reaching twenty weeks are very much 'wanted' children.

*'Perhaps I wouldn't go back and say I'd rather not have had
congenital heart disease.'*

Many young people who have had operations say they are proud
of their scars – they appreciate that their early troubles have made
them the person they are now happy to be. Their survival has
brought a resilience, perhaps even a sense that the worst thing that
will ever happen to them is already in their past. But this particular
quote comes from Diana, whose insights we should take very seriously. She knows more than anyone about facing life and death
with incapacitating heart disease, and she has a window into other
people's lives because she is an astute psychologist.

Diana was born in the 1950s with 'congenitally corrected transposition' and a Ventricular Septal Defect (VSD). No surgery was
offered and by her teenage years she was blue with Eisenmenger's
syndrome. In the chapter about pregnancy, we encountered her
as an undergraduate facing a decision about being sterilized. Her
limited stamina made her bookish, but that did mean that she got
an excellent degree. A PhD followed, then some post-doctoral
work and a move into clinical psychology. Through her thirties she
became increasingly exhausted, hardly able to walk even a short
distance, working in the National Health Service as a consultant
psychologist. She recognizes in her former self the determination
shared by some people whose life is on a short fuse – doing what
people do when they cannot take life for granted. She married,
and that too gave her a reason for living.

Having resisted, in her forties she accepted a wheelchair and
found it 'bloody wonderful'; she was able to get out to the cinema. Likewise, accepting oxygen therapy: 'Why hadn't I done
that earlier?' Incapacity Benefit was 'definitely a win'. As a psychologist, she had strategies for managing her own anger – 'Set
boundaries on moaning', 'Look deliberately at the pros and cons
of victimhood'. This is a 'bloody-minded' woman with a fund

of black humour stories, but even she sometimes felt like giving up completely.

Having confounded everyone by living into her forties, she was assessed for a heart and lung transplant. Her Eisenmenger's* meant that neither a heart-only nor a lung-only transplant would be enough. Heart and lung transplants are rare (only one was performed in the UK in 2014–15) – if split, the precious donor organs could benefit two or even three people. Diana hated hospitals, she hated the 'can't guarantee . . . ' drift of all the conversations with the transplant team; all the details seemed a package of horror. It helped that a transplant would either work or she would be dead.

A physician she trusted gave her a pep-talk about making her choice one way or the other, and then being wholehearted. Terror of dying was not what pushed her into a decision – she was very matter-of-fact about death, but she really didn't want to go on living long and being so disabled. She was listed for the operation, and told to try to stay well while she waited. During this uncertain time she could think ahead. She wanted to feel that others would be okay, whatever happened. She organized her funeral and dealt with her will. She had time to talk to her mother and to her husband about his future should 'death do us part'. There were quite a lot of tears.

Then, after an eight-month wait, her call came. Her donor was a young woman who had died of a brain haemorrhage and whose devastated family had been generous. It took much of the next year for Diana to get over the transplant operation. The medication regime – even breathing and moving – needed to be mastered. That was thirteen years ago.

Diana has since buried her own mother – such a natural thing that neither of them had dreamed she would ever do. She is back

* Reminder: Eisenmenger's syndrome is an umbrella term for patients with 'high blood pressure' in their lung circuit, due to an uncorrected heart condition.

at work. Professionally, Diana has had a privileged view of other people's inner worlds and has listened as her patients have negotiated their own health troubles and disappointments. As a lifetime student of the human condition, she recognizes how we all want the best parts of other people's lives but not their whole reality. Her sense is that life as a 'normal' person would not necessarily have been any happier than hers had been. She still thinks 'Oh bugger' sometimes, but when I asked her what she might change, she said cautiously, 'Perhaps I wouldn't go back and say I'd rather not have had congenital heart disease'. Who better to know?

> 'You are not choosing life and death here; that is already decided. You are choosing who is going to be with her and how she will be loved and supported when the time arrives.'

The scenario here is a contemporary intensive care unit (ICU); the quote comes from a particular doctor, but this conversation could happen in any fortnight in any busy cardiac surgical unit. The child's parents have been sitting at her bedside for days, probably weeks, possibly months. There have been good days, but many setbacks, and though the doctors are not at the end of their resources, they are wondering if the next foreseeable intrusion might possibly not be a good idea.

Current children's ICUs are unrecognizable from their counterparts in the 1950s. They are run by specialist doctors who use an arsenal of drugs and devices, inconceivable fifty years ago. Racks of syringes at each bedside infuse medications for stimulating this, quietening that or making war on germs. Lungs can be supported with ventilators and kidneys substituted with dialysis machines; it is even possible to take over the work of the heart and lungs completely – for a while. Intensivists are extremely good at keeping babies alive, but sometimes they struggle to actually make them better. Their increasing expertise has meant that most children pass through ICUs more quickly than previously, but a few are left in a parlous state, dependent too long on the machinery surrounding them. In previous years, these children would probably have died. The longer the stay in ICU, the higher the chance of dying in hospital, and if the child survives, long-stay is also a marker for later difficulties with learning, memory, language development and other skills. These are generalities; it is difficult to predict what a particular child's future will be.

The culture of most ICUs is for doctors to be cheerleaders for the parents sitting at the bedside day by day, offering hope and encouragement through the setbacks that are so common in that environment. For most families their optimism is justified and their child follows 'Plan A', and is discharged to an ordinary ward after some days to start getting on with his life. But when problems drag on it can be hard for both parents and doctors to change gear, to even talk about what 'Plans B or C' might look like. For a child with a long ICU stay related to a heart that cannot be passably repaired, death in hospital must be one of the possible futures that they face.

Apart from instances of terrible brain damage, a child's death does not usually come after some life-or-death decision that involves 'pulling the plug' on a ventilator. Much more often it follows a decision not to try another round of antibiotics or not to put a child back on a ventilator or not to pump on her chest if her heart stops. Agreeing some limit on intensive care for a child is visibly gruelling for parents. When a child is lying immobile, invaded by multiple tubes, it can be difficult to intuit whether she is suffering or not; on a ventilator, sedated and paralysed with drugs, obvious awareness rarely breaks through. By the time these conversations happen, the family is often exhausted and finds it hard to reconcile the doctors' apparently gloomy change of heart with their previous assured confidence. Some become angry, refusing to stop believing wholeheartedly in the happy ending of 'Plan A' – it is very difficult to talk to parents who do not even permit the word 'death' to be spoken aloud. Some forcefully demand that 'no limits' are placed on attempts to save their child's life, but in truth not all problems have a solution. These children may die with the team pumping on their chests, more tubes, more blood; yet parents and some doctors may feel that by doing these things their 'duty' is done.

Other families who have been silently rehearsing their child's death in their minds are grateful for an intensivist's offer to talk. Hopefully the doctor will manage to avoid saying 'There is nothing more we can do' – because the caring part of medicine goes on to the end. Sadly, some families are too numb to see this as a valuable time. If they are lucky, there will be someone in the unit who believes that treatment aimed at improving the quality of death is not futile. They will help parents organize the things they want to happen – the people who are to be present, the mementos they want to keep. People have taken photographs, made sketches, handprints, footprints, special boxes of keepsakes as they prepare to lose their child. Occasionally the child improves, at other times she dies – either way, being part of the planning is usually valuable for families. Taking some control gives the people left behind a chance to show their love.*

'Death alone is certain, the time of death is uncertain.'

This is not a quote but a sort of koan, used over the centuries by teachers from Buddha to the commanders of Roman soldiers. It challenges our illusion of permanence. The Roman commander requires of his troops that while they live, they fight. The meditation teacher reminds the student that every breath takes him nearer to his last breath. Many of us manage to potter through life

---

* Such evidence as exists suggests that parents who manage to take some control over a child's death 'adjust better' in its aftermath.

for many years never making the connection between these man-
ifestly true words and our familiar and apparently reliable bodies.
But people whose hearts have already wavered once often feel the
urgency of the koan. Telling others in her survivors' Facebook
group that she was going back to college, Sarah said, 'I'm going
to *carpe* the hell out of my *diem* and finish the degree I've always
wanted'; two months later she was dead.

This feisty attitude is born of something profound. Over the
months of listening to 'ordinary' people as they talked to me about
how their hearts have influenced their perspectives, I have come to
wonder why we seem so addicted to admiring only 'extraordinary'
achievements. We met Wendy qualifying as a social worker in the
chapter on growing up. Her stamina was always marginal and it
took unconditional resolve to qualify and then simply hold down a
job as a social worker. By twenty-five years after her big operation,
she was experiencing heart rhythm problems which sapped her
energy and she had to stop working. Back in the 1980s, transplantation had been talked of as her eventual 'last resort' – the doctors
were pessimistic that the 'Fontan circulation' would last long-term.
Through her teens and early twenties, a later transplant was still
talked of as part of the game-plan, but two decades later, when she
actually came to ask about its timing, people started back-pedalling,
citing 'problems' from her previous surgery, antibodies in her blood
from previous transfusions, lack of donors . . .*

---

* In the interim, it emerged that transplants for 'end-stage' operated congenital
heart disease carried a higher risk in the early aftermath of the surgery than
the much more common transplants for 'heart muscle disease'. That said, if
the congenital patients survived their transplants, they tended to do at least as
well as the others. The paradox emerges that while a transplant may still give
a congenital heart patient their best chance of a longer life, the donated heart
may 'live longer' if it were put into someone else.

It seemed that a lifeline had been withdrawn and for a while a 'grey mist' descended. She talked both to her precious cardiologist and her wonderful surgeon (both long retired) about whether or not to embark on a major revision of her imperfect Fontan 'plumbing' or perhaps plead for a transplant. Using virtual networks, Wendy took care to consult other survivors of early Fontan operations from all over the world. With or without re-plumbing* or transplantation, none seemed very much better than she was herself.

Wendy thought through the different gambles on offer but eventually baulked at the possibility of being on a trolley going into an operation and perhaps never seeing her family again. She decided against any further surgery. Through social media she has met several other 'Fontans' of what she calls 'her generation'. Last year she and a friend travelled together to a funeral of another of their virtual group – the full horse-drawn-carriage-final-journey. 'Bye; see you in a few years,' they agreed.

After years of driving herself to achieve, Wendy is taking time to smell the roses. More than thirty years after her Fontan operation she sends occasional emails to her cardiologist with photos of 'Wendy with a rock-star' or 'Wendy in Tiananmen Square', as she works through her bucket list with the help of her family. It hurts her to think that some people in her situation have not thrown themselves at life.

If focusing the mind on 'death may come today' is a fast-track path to realization, a betting Buddhist teacher would probably wager on people with an Implantable Cardioverter Defibrillator being the first to reach enlightenment. When their hearts' rhythms misbehave in dangerous ways they lose consciousness, often in

---

* This would have involved a conversion to a Total Cavo Pulmonary Connection, a Fontan-type circuit engineered to minimize obstruction in the route to the lungs.

the middle of everyday life – they may simply fall down in a dead faint in the kitchen, in a lift or on the football field. Without the technology in their hearts, that would be the end – 'sudden cardiac death'. To some, that may sound like the perfect way to go, but their 'box' senses the rhythm changes and – usually when the patient is already unconscious on the floor – it delivers a shock sufficient for the patient's whole body to jerk. All being well, one shock is sufficient to revert the tricky rhythm and within a few coordinated heartbeats consciousness returns, the patient thinks 'Did I faint?' and then remembers . . . Mostly, patients both love and hate their 'guardian angel'; being shocked can unleash 'fury and resentment' against the unfairness of their lot, but it also reinforces their will to live. Which of us would be unchanged by living with such a reminder that 'Death alone is certain, the time of death is uncertain'?

What is most personal is most universal

This is the paradox experienced by the people who are left behind – and those people are many. The babies, children and adults who have died of their congenital heart disease are far outnumbered by those who loved them and watched them die; and are then left to grieve. Babies, children and adults all leave different-shaped voids for their brothers, sisters, fathers, mothers, husbands, wives and friends.

At the funeral ceremony, the one who has died is lapped in love and their family surrounded with sympathy. But then a coffin goes into a musty, damp and surprisingly deep hole and everyone gradually begins to accelerate away from that moment at a different speed. Spouses don't want to pull their partners under, brothers and sisters go quiet – for everyone, the path feels solitary and very personal. It takes a poet to convey that the journey of bereavement is universal too – and we have a poet to speak for us. Rebecca Goss chronicles birth, life, death and grief in her book of poetry about her daughter who died of Ebstein's anomaly at sixteen months of age. Towards the end of the collection, she writes to her new baby:

> *Taking you there*
> Parked up by the dunes, we tucked you
> into your pram, pulled on our wellington boots.
>
> We pushed towards the sea, lifted you
> over the final rise, dropped onto pebbles
>
> and the deserted beach. For a time we just stood there,
> facing the spray, before deciding the best way
>
> was to free you from straps and carry you in.
> Your father carried you tight against his coat,
>
> his spare hand locked in mine.
> We waded forward, into the same cold pull
>
> that took the ashes of your sister,
> and lifted you above our heads.
>
> Your baby's face was blustered by the wind
> and we cried beneath your gasping laughs
>
> as waves splashed inside our boots.
> The unimaginable thought of you, last time
>
> we were here, when we turned our backs and left her,
> eddying in the tug. Ashore, I pushed the pram
>
> but your father carried you back to the car,
> unwilling to give up your squirming limbs.

19
What's new? (Besides innovation)

Hawick is a small town in the Scottish Borders, famous for knitwear and rugby; Louise was born there in 1970. By six months of age she was noticeably blue and some Edinburgh doctors recognized that she had Transposition of the Great Arteries (TGA). The 'Great Arteries' are the aorta (body) and pulmonary (lung) arteries and the 'Transposition' simply means that they come off the wrong ventricles (pumping chambers). The heart being otherwise normal, this means that the blue blood is pumped out to the body and the red blood to the lungs – a very unpromising arrangement that fewer than half of babies survive for even three months without treatment.

At that time, there was no radical surgery for this condition available locally, so with their conspicuously blue eighteen-month-old baby in their laps, Louise's parents took the train to London. Her father was a wool-sorter of modest means and this was his first trip south. The local Rotary Club had donated a bit towards the family's costs and they stayed with a relative, travelling thirty stops into central London on the Underground to see their daughter. Between visits to Louise's ward, they drifted around Bloomsbury where one morning they turned a corner and bumped into a local hero from home – an international rugby player. 'What were they doing in London?' Hearing their tale, he pulled out his wallet – 'Have some lunch on me' – a gesture of Scottish solidarity.*

Louise had a Mustard operation, which over the course of a few hours changed her from being unmistakably blue to pleasingly pink. (The Mustard operation leaves the great arteries wrongly connected, but switches the blue and red blood's routes as the veins arrive back to the heart; thus the venous return sorts out the blue/red issues but leaves the right (wrong) ventricle serving the body's circulation.) Her parents took the train north with their beautiful, blonde and photogenic baby, back to a brief celebrity in the local newspapers and her right (wrong) ventricle has provided the pumping power for her body circulation through her schooling and later her busy working life and a pregnancy. For the next forty years, Louise had no cause to worry about her heart.

I have present-day Louise to thank for opening a window into a world I might never otherwise have appreciated, one that I believe will be more crucially progressive than all the eye-catching innovations of artificial heart technology or stem-cell remedies. From their particular place in the history of the treatment of congenital heart disease, I think Louise and her 'friends' have lessons to teach patients and doctors alike – lessons about knowledge, solidarity and *joie de vivre*.

Some background about TGA. It is the commonest plumbing problem to make a newborn baby look unmistakably blue.

---

* This was Hugh McLeod a.k.a. the 'Hawick Hardman', a Scottish prop forward described by a colleague as 'harder than teak'. In his 2014 obituary, an opponent remembered how delighted he had been to be lining up against the legend and telling McLeod as they ran out of the tunnel that he was looking forward to learning from him. In the first scrum, the youngster put his hand on the ground as he tried to position himself against the Hawick front row and McLeod duly stood hard on it, with the immortal words: 'Here endeth the first lesson.' Not a soppy man.

During the 1950s, some surgeons would attempt a sort of 'smash and grab' operation* to make a hole in the atrial septum; when successful, this allowed the blue and red blood to mingle in the atrial 'collecting-chambers' and transformed the amounts of oxygen reaching the body from unsurvivably low to survivable-but-very-blue levels. Later, these holes were made using a balloon, manipulated in the X-ray department, up through a vein and used to rip the wall between the atrial chambers; this is the procedure Jai had in the chapter about the perils of being born and Louise herself had in Edinburgh. After these temporizing interventions, babies grew to be spectacularly blue children presenting a 'now what' challenge to the teams looking after them.

In the late 1950s, there were one or two attempts to rejoin the 'Great Arteries' correctly (precursors of the so-called 'arterial switch' operation), but the surgery involved handling the 2mm-diameter vessels supplying the heart itself. The operations needed to be carried out on newborn babies, and experience and equipment were simply not up to the task; all the babies died. Instead, surgeons Senning (in Sweden) and Mustard (in Canada) came up with similar operations that bear their different names. Both operations are notorious for their origami-like challenge to the surgeon's 3-dimensional sense. In the 'Mustard operation', he cuts away the original wall between the two collecting chambers before sewing in some fabric to make a new partition. The fabric forms a baffle that diverts the red blood as it arrives at the back of the heart (from the lungs) directing it forwards into the front ('right') ventricle; the veins carrying blue blood (from the body) are funnelled in a chicane behind the baffle into the

---

* This was the Blalock-Hanlon operation. Other approaches included cutting the right pulmonary veins away from the left atrium and implanting them onto the right atrium or cutting the inferior vena cava away from the right atrium and implanting it onto the left atrium. The Blalock-Hanlon operation proved the least worst of these alternatives.

back ('left') ventricle. This 'venous switch' leaves the children pink without doing anything radical about the primary problem of the wrongly connected arteries. The Mustard and Senning operations could wait until the first couple of *years* of life, provided someone had earlier stabilized the child by making a satisfactory hole in the wall between the atria.

The very first child to have a baffle operation died after his 'successful' surgery. In 1956, there was no ventilator to support such a small baby and the doomed little boy could not breathe satisfactorily on his own because of his massive chest incision. But TGA is common and babies who would inevitably die without surgery were arriving in the large specialist units every week. Learning case-by-case, by the late 1960s the teams that had mastered the Mustard or Senning operations, and had learned how to take over a baby's breathing safely with a ventilator after their surgery, were recording big business.

By the 1970s, the operations devised by Drs Mustard and Senning had completely reversed the fortunes of babies born with TGA. From an everyday point of view, surviving children were almost indistinguishable from normal. But there was genuine concern that they might run into heart failure later in life because their operations were not 'corrective' in the sense of putting right the 'wrong' connections of the great arteries; their new circulations delivered blue and red blood to the right place, but their left and right ventricles were doing each other's work and it was uncertain how long the right ventricle would manage to sustain the body's circulation before eventually caving in. As it happens, there is a rare but naturally occurring defect called 'congenitally corrected transposition' in which the heart's connections correspond exactly to the Mustard operation's in terms of blood flow,*

---

* In congenitally corrected transposition (a.k.a. 'double discordance'), the *left* atrium is connected to the *right* ventricle which is connected to the *aorta*. The

so we could anticipate that Mustard survivors might encounter the same long-term complications that we know congenitally corrected transposition patients come to suffer. Patients with this condition are born with their right ventricles pumping blood to their bodies, yet can remain well for decades without any surgery. But evolution did not 'build' right ventricles to do this job. By the age of sixty, over half the people with congenitally corrected transposition are in real trouble with heart failure. This concern for the long term was the impetus to try once again to accomplish the more anatomically corrective arterial switch operation that had first been attempted in the 1950s. The first successful arterial switch operation was carried out in Brazil in 1975. At its outset, the 'switch' seemed a surgical tour-de-force. Besides sorting out the two main 'pipes' coming off the heart, the two coronary arteries that feed the heart itself had to be individually transferred from the old to the new aorta – of newborn babies.

When the first switch survival was announced at a big inter-national meeting in Los Angeles in 1976, the surgical audience was thrilled. The concept was recognized as a turning point – though when you read the small print of that key announcement, only one of the seven babies operated left hospital alive. As usual in medical papers, we learn none of the names of the six casualties, nor of the lone survivor. We have already met Simon in an earlier chapter, explaining why he does not plan to marry. He first got in touch to tell me his family's story. His sister had been born a few years before him with Transposition and had died after a Mustard operation in 1971. So when he was born with the same condition,* the local team suggested that his parents take their son elsewhere

right atrium is connected to the *left* ventricle, which is connected to the *pulmon-ary artery*. This circuit requires the right ventricle to push blood around the body – and its tricuspid valve not to leak at this high pressure.

★ It is unusual for Transposition to recur in a family.

to see if a London unit could do better. There, Simon had an arterial switch operation in 1976. As I spoke to Simon, I realized this date was quite early in the history of switch surgery and, after a little detective work, established that he had had the second ever switch operation in England. After I had sent him the publication documenting this, his email reply read: 'WOW. I am tingling. That is so strange to read, it's about me!!!' Any doctor working in the paediatric cardiology trade would immediately recognize the name of the surgeon who did that operation,* but I think it is a shame that patients rarely know their part in history.

Over the next decade, the arterial switch operation became established as the go-to option for babies born with TGA. There was a tough learning curve, because the steps of transferring the coronary arteries from the old to the new aorta are very fiddly. The surgeon needs to work with magnifying loupes and fine fil-ament suture materials. At the beginning, the new operation was the province of elite surgeons; it required a lot of experience and a good spatial sense of how all the vessels were to sit together at the end of the repair. Increasing the stress, this learning on the part of some surgeons was going on in parallel to other surgeons con-tinuing to do the Mustard or Senning operations – and for some years the older baffle operations were producing more short-term survivors. But the surgeons persevered with the more 'corrective' concept of the arterial switch in the belief that it would prove a better investment for the adulthood of babies born with TGA. Gradually the steps of the arterial switch were standardized and – much as a daunting recipe promoted by a celebrity chef eventually reaches the recipe books of ordinary kitchens – the arterial switch operation has entered the repertoire of every children's heart sur-geon. In 2014 there were no operative deaths in any of the 145 British babies who had an arterial switch operation in the first

---

* This was Donald Ross.

month of life – which is remarkable considering that their hearts are the size of a fat strawberry and their coronary arteries no thicker than a strand of vermicelli.

We cannot yet be absolutely sure that the arterial switch has won the battle for the adult future of babies born with TGA – though this is very likely. While Louise and her 'kindred' patients who had a Mustard procedure are hitting middle age, even the earliest switch patients are significantly younger. These switch survivors have already had some surgery on their coronary arteries but have not yet entered the age group that begins to get trouble with the sort of coronary artery disease in which plaques of cholesterol-type material start blocking people's blood vessels. We already know that not every switch survivor has perfect coronary arteries, so it is impossible to be completely reassuring that some may not have trouble ahead.*

So where does this leave patients like Louise who have had an operation that history has left behind? Surgeons these days would struggle to do a Mustard or Senning procedure – most have never even seen one done. Many younger cardiologists are also unfamiliar with the workings of these whacky hearts. Mustard and Senning survivors are all now between twenty-something and fifty-something years old, corresponding to the first and last wave of the baffle operations. We already know that some of them are running into exactly the problems that were anticipated in the 1960s and 1970s. Some of their right ventricles (and tricuspid valves which are not ideally built for a job in a high-pressure circuit) are beginning to struggle, the patients becoming tired and breathless as their hearts fail to deliver as much pump-work as previously. They are also prone to heart-rhythm problems related to all the stitching in their atria and to clogging-up or leaking of their baffle channels.

---

* Fortunately, doctors are quite good at treating coronary artery problems these days.

When I met Louise, she was forty-five and was just getting over her very first heart-related setback. We had arranged to meet in the foyer of a London hotel, but I did not recognize her initially. I'm not sure what I had expected, but somehow I was not looking out for the sort of stylish, full-of-life woman who was waiting there. We spent a happy couple of hours chatting, drinking tea and drifting around Bloomsbury like her parents had done years before. Louise showed me a photo with her teenage daughter – they could have been sisters. After we parted, I wondered about my earlier confusion. As doctors, we see patients in hospital wards and clinics: in 'our' territory. Working in a children's service, I also say goodbye to them when they are in their mid teens. Though I should have known better, I realized that I had unconsciously stuck with the image of a 'patient' as looking passive, a bit downtrodden, a little needy, the out-patient-waiting-room look. Doctors, I have to tell you that Louise and others I have met out 'in the wild' are not like that at all! She was a live-wire, on top of things; *she* was helping *me*. I am embarrassed to admit my misconception – but it was only my first lesson.

The second lesson was even more humbling. Before we said goodbye, Louise offered to 'introduce' me to her Facebook group. For my generation, Facebook often gets a bad rap, and I was not immune to that. I accepted her invitation but was completely unprepared to have my prejudices overturned so comprehensively. The 'Mustard and Senning Survivors Facebook Group' is closed – you don't get to look at the 'conversations' unless you are a member, and virtually all the members have survived Mustard or Senning surgery.

At first I felt voyeuristic. There are over 700 in the group, spread over four continents. No single doctor or hospital service can begin to compete with the tonnage of life experience of this out-of-the-ordinary circulation that this community hold. Their conversations are in English, which the Scandinavians, Spanish and

Germans seem to manage effortlessly. The moderators from within the group keep an eye on the chat with a combination of firmness and lightness of touch that seems to be well respected. One-to-one chats can happen entirely in private and particular friendships have clearly evolved. As new people join the group, they are plainly delighted to have finally found others who are sharing their very particular lifeboat.

Just how representative the members of the group are of the worldwide Mustard and Senning community is difficult to tell. They certainly seem to cover the whole spectrum of ages of Mustard and Senning survivors. Many give a 'shout' when their birthday or surgery-anniversary comes around; the oldest I have noticed was recently fifty-seven. Some members have had a clear run since their operation with no drama or further surgery. Others have had a tough time – young people who have lived with heart failure for many years. From time to time, straw polls ask: Have you got a pacemaker? / Have they treated a baffle-leak? / Have you been told not to get pregnant?; it appears that the whole spectrum of problems (and lack of problems) is represented among their number.

Posts to the group contain a good proportion of banter. 'Getting to know you' is helped by 'Show me a picture' of your pet/your home-town/your tattoos. Or 'It's Friday, tell us a joke.' Weddings and newborn babies make for happy pictures and warm congratulations. In the face of all the 'trivia' my Facebook cynicism oddly faded away. Just as the telephone changed the reach of friendship, social media has brought something positive and new – even to medicine. These people are not tied together by real encounters (mostly, they have never met), yet are genuine friends – and impressively so. Across time zones, they can simply say they are having a tough day and be heard. 'Thanks everyone, nobody else "gets it"' is a common comment. They can whinge about a crass doctor or a chaotic clinic and get replies that remind them of the funny side. But they can also talk about sensitive anxieties, perhaps hearts and sex: 'Here's a question for the boys', or 'What have you told your kids?'

As a doctor, I'm fascinated to read through dozens of responses to 'If there was one thing that you could change about yourself, what would it be?' (some would choose to change their hearts, but not a majority). Or 'What were you/your parents told about why were you born with Transposition?' (stories about mothers' contact with pills, insecticides, cleaning products, radiation exposure or German Measles came back).* Members ask for recommendations of a good doctor in their vicinity; they moan if they meet a clueless one at a clinic.

Understandably, people post questions to the group when they have an imminent concern. And what a resource! 'I'm pregnant and seeing my obstetrician for the first time; is there anything particular I should ask them?' Within twenty-four hours there are ten pertinent, practical responses, born of personal experience. Or 'I don't understand the jargon on my exercise test report' (attaching a readable photo of the document). I can tell that some members really know their stuff, because back comes an authoritative explanation of the numbers. Or 'How bad do you have to be before they consider you for a transplant?' Bouncing back come replies from people who have been listed for transplantation, people who have been turned down for a transplant and people who are living with a heart transplant. 'If our right ventricles aren't great, why can't they just do a switch operation on us?' (In return come well-researched replies: 'In principle, yes it's possible – though not easy; in practice, the risks are very high', accompanied by links to the medical articles that document the difficulties.) 'Do you have nightmares?', 'Does drug X give you migraines?', 'How long before you went back to work after a baffle stent?', 'They are talking about

---

* The 'correct' answer even now is: 'We still don't really know.'

bi-ventricular pacing – good or what?' Questions large and small receive helpful answers.

It is not all good news. Members' families alert the group to deaths among their number. The condolences sent back are heart-felt, flowers go to funerals. These friends died young; they had been surrounded by people who loved them, they may have had children – and they were travelling a similar route to the others in the group. The mood is sombre for a while.

Honestly, I am in awe of these people. I admire how they support each other and how they conduct their lives with their eyes open. Sarah is thirty-something and by her own account has had a fairly smooth run through her post-Mustard-operation life to date. She is an academic librarian with a PhD and enough geeky competence and mediation skills to be one of the administrators that keep the Mustard and Senning Survivors group so engaged and running smoothly. We discussed its recipe for success. The members are all adults, all plainly 'survivors' and at least twenty-something years old; this in itself means that they have a lot of life experience and a well-developed sense of proportion. Though there are some 'friends and relations' in the group – including a few mothers – they mainly keep quiet; scanning some other congenital heart forums, the dread and terror that mothers of young children sometimes express can feel contagious. It may help that their Mustard and Senning Survivors niche is quite specific; though they share many issues with people who have come through other congenital heart surgeries, the complications they experience are quite particular to their funky hearts. The collective knowledge of the group has gradually accumulated – a few individuals take trouble to delve into the formal medical literature to understand other people's problems. Finally, it may be an advantage that the group does not exist under the auspices of some other organization, for example a national support group, a charity or a particular hospital. Many of these have websites, often with slightly different agendas – information-giving, advocacy, money-raising or even (dare I say it) advertising. Each of these serves a worthwhile purpose, but their mission statements are not primarily the kind of person-to-person support that is so valuable for people in an exceptional situation.

The group grew from small beginnings. In early 2009 the Mustard-repaired heart of a father of two living in New Zealand* was getting to the end of its useful life. On the waiting list for a transplant and with 'not much else to do other than research TGA', he corralled the few people he knew with Mustard or Senning operations into a new Facebook group. A combination of word of mouth and internet blunderings have accumulated the 700+ 'insiders' that we see today; many people are first drawn in after chancing across a link when looking for information on the web when they were having a rough time. Sarah's sense is that people dip in and out of contact as their needs arise. Some may post a question or respond to someone else's query if they have something particular to offer. Others skim through the stories and absorb impressions that gradually add to their grasp of their own situation without leaving any trace of their visits to the pages. It is helpful that they can work at their own speed because the news is not always easy. With so many members, people are posting from hospital beds every week and major surgery, transplant sagas and deaths occasionally feature. Sarah herself has hesitated to visit the Facebook page when she is apprehensive about what she would read, but now regards her part in facilitating the group as 'giving back' to the whole community.

---

* This was Stuart Watson, by then already a veteran of supporting kids, teens, adults and families with CHD. The group fulfilled a dream of bringing together survivors for mutual support. 'I just didn't know how. Facebook gave me my How and the twenty or so friends who initially joined me helped me turn the dream into a reality.' As the group grew, its 'rules of engagement' clarified, other 'administrators' were co-opted and with secure foundations the group took on a life of its own. An amazing achievement.

'I find the gig at turns humbling, joyous, terrifying and comforting. Sometimes all in the span of a day.'

I want to make the case that virtual networks of patients have more potential to improve the lot of congenital heart disease survivors than any of the high-tech medical innovations that are on the horizon. Undoubtedly, some patients will have years added to their lives by transplants or artificial hearts or clever pacemakers or new drugs – but *information* has the potential to save lives too. What is so interesting to me as a doctor is that the medical profession does not control these virtual communities.

Of all 'categories' of patients, those with congenital heart disease are probably the ones who most need to take charge of their relationship with the medical community. For a start, these people aim to live with the hearts they were born with for many decades – much longer than any single professional lifetime. Long-term relationships between particular patients and particular doctors look 'like marriage without the romance', but over a patient's whole lifetime, one or other party to the marriage will move away, retire or otherwise 'divorce'. Information that should get passed along can easily get lost in any disruption, unless the patients themselves keep track. Second, the branch of medicine they depend on is fast-moving; this means that doctors' advice given in good faith in one century may turn out to be mistaken in the next. ('Off you go, you are cured', 'You can always have a transplant when your circulation eventually fails' and 'Sennings are unlikely to survive to thirty'* are all statements made to people featuring in this book, and all have turned out to be materially wrong.) Finally, heart centres do not take responsibility for tracking their patients over

---

* For a thirty-five-year-old new member of the Mustard and Senning Facebook group, having this statement refuted must have cheered her up a lot. (The original statement was made in the era when doctors were bargaining over the move to the arterial switch operation.)

their lifetimes; it is the patients themselves who must hustle to keep contact with their doctors.

We believe that there are hundreds of thousands of people worldwide with childhood scars on their chests who are completely adrift from expert follow-up.* The older ones lost contact in their teens before useful adult services even existed; younger people may simply lose touch as they move around the country, often in the honeymoon period of feeling well and getting on with their lives. Without knowing it, some of them are vulnerable to the insidious changes that go on to 'bankrupt' their hearts 'gradually then suddenly'. People with long gaps between visits (sometimes decades) tend to arrive back at hospitals in crisis, so getting former patients into timely contact with a competent doctor may be a complete game-changer for their futures. Like many conditions, heart problems are best caught while they are brewing and before they cause symptoms.

But how is this return to the fold actually to come about? A 'worried well' adult survivor detached from follow-up might ask their own family doctor about the implications of their previous surgery. They could be unusually lucky, but honestly – given that adult congenital heart disease is such an esoteric branch of medicine – they might more usefully turn to Dr Google. Type 'Mustard', 'Fallot' or 'coarctation' into a search engine and you

---

* Because comprehensive lists of patients who had early surgery are hard to make in retrospect and because death certification does not link up with medical records in most countries, there is therefore a knowledge vacuum about the shortfall in numbers of patients being looked after to current standards – perhaps 50 per cent. This also makes it difficult to claim that specialist follow-up adds years to the lives of congenital heart patients – though it almost certainly does. Handovers from childhood to adult clinics are better (though not perfectly) organized now.

have hours of browsing ahead.* Medical staff may bluster about the (un)dependability of internet information but – to be candid – the knowledge that most doctors carry about these topics would be limited to how to spell the words. As in every other field, some internet information is rubbish, but Wikipedia entries are evidently drafted by medical specialists. Also, many bona fide stakeholders in the enterprise of congenital heart disease have an internet presence: websites of hospital services and charities promoting research all provide different sorts of information. Advocacy groups are a good source of summaries written in natural language rather than medical jargon. Some of it is a little dry and dusty – these organizations are telling the reader stuff, not promoting a conversation. The pictures they paint of life with congenital heart disease are often a little varnished; the photos are resolutely upbeat.

To get a less sanitized image and some real-life advice about their heart, a patient's browsing must reach one of the many support groups. Some welcome people of all ages, diagnoses and experiences, others are focused in some way – by age, diagnosis, region, even gender. Each has its own character and rules of engagement; amounts of traffic vary enormously. Some defer frequently to doctors to answer medical questions. Others have chosen to educate themselves. A really enterprising non-medic can access medical journals on the internet where many papers are 'open source' – meaning that if you can find them, you can read them. Understanding them is more difficult, but some 'expert patients' come to know a lot about the small domain of medicine relevant to their condition. Support groups are very open-minded about picking up naive questions that people might hesitate to ask a doctor, and it only needs a few knowledgeable people in a

---

* Searches are difficult for adult survivors who do not know the name either of their condition or their operation; their parents may be dead or have forgotten.

community to raise everyone else's understanding of a condition they have in common. Some advocacy groups even keep a close eye on the surgical results of surgical centres in their own country to be ready with enquiries from parents about where to go for a second opinion.

All support groups know the value of finding a doctor with the right range of experience; 'generalist' doctors offer breadth, 'specialist' doctors offer depth. As the medical profession begins to lose the monopoly on medical knowledge, the doctor–patient relationship starts to shift; how this plays out varies from one consulting room to the next. However, if by their grasp of the issues patients come to contribute to their own care and influence the services they rely on, this success will be in no small part due to the maturation of internet support groups.

If someone finds a support group aimed at their own diagnosis, like the Mustard and Senning Survivors group serves people born with TGA before the mid 1980s, they have also found a resource that adds quality to their lives – friends who 'get it' in a way that we who have no experience of their journey through life cannot do. I am a fan and asked Louise's group for some final words. I am too embarrassed to list their 'Ten things dopey doctors have said to me' but, to give you some takeaway messages and a flavour of what they have to offer, here are:

Ten things not to say to a person with congenital heart disease
- Can't you just get a heart transplant?
- Your scar is gross.
- You're just used to being coddled, if you pushed yourself harder you could do it/more.
- You're a Miracle! God must have saved you to do Something Special.
- Does that mean you will drop down dead one day?
- When will the doctors fix you?

- Don't worry you should be just fine.
- You haven't done anything all day, how could you be tired.
- Really? I guess you could go back to the doctor; even though they have years of education, medical school, etc. they make mistakes.
- I know just what you're going through.

★ ★ ★

Looking back at the last century, the drive to advance the treatment of congenital heart disease was the exclusive province of doctors (often surgeons) and researchers and their funders. Early patients and their families, while not exactly commodities, were not agents. Yet like the 'Poor Bloody Infantry' of the First World War, they played a crucial part in the campaign. Unfortunately, if there had been medals for their services (which there were not) many would have been posthumous. Yet every operation, successful or not, teaches its team a lesson and every current surgical patient is the beneficiary of those lessons.

When we look at the prospect for further advances in the current century, the traditional, medically based agencies are still delivering innovation – implantable valves, stem-cell grafts, mechanical devices. These are mostly treatments for end-stage disease that everyone hopes that few will need. But if we gauge medical progress by its capacity to improve the length and quality of the lives of many patients, there is a new kid on the block. The new agent for change is the power of patients acting together. Surfing on the power of the internet to put people in touch with each other, support groups move information around; they put the right information in front of the right people at the time when they need it and give them courage to act on it. And, like no other community, they show their supporters how to live. If there were an award for our era's 'best medical innovation', I would nominate patient support groups.

APPENDIX

Schematic diagrams help some people understand the mechanics of the heart's blood flow, though they struggle to convey its 3D structure. These figures show the circuits of the normal heart in a child (where the lungs provide the oxygen) and in the fetus (where oxygen is picked up from the placenta). Also shown are the abnormal blood flows caused by some of the defects encountered in several chapters.

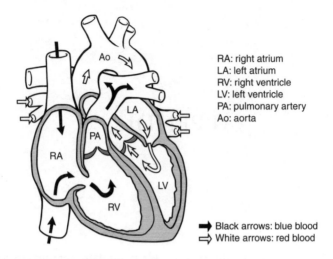

RA: right atrium
LA: left atrium
RV: right ventricle
LV: left ventricle
PA: pulmonary artery
Ao: aorta

➡ Black arrows: blue blood
⇨ White arrows: red blood

Fig. 1: The normal heart

In the normal heart, blue blood from the body arrives in the right atrium (before being pumped out to the lungs), and red blood from the lungs arrives in the left atrium (before being pumped out to the body).

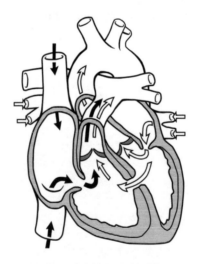

Fig. 2: Ventricular Septal Defect (VSD)

This shows a VSD with a 'left to right shunt'. Red blood is crossing over from the left ventricle into the right ventricle, and mixing with the blue blood there. (If the lung resistance goes up, the shunt could reverse, with blue blood reaching the left ventricle and hence the aorta.)

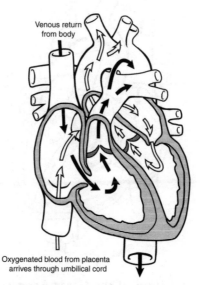

Fig. 3: Heart in the fetus

In the fetus, the lungs are squashed with hardly any blood flow through them. Blood pumped out from the right ventricle crosses a duct which joins the pulmonary artery to the aorta. Oxygenated blood arriving from the placenta tends to stream through a hole between the atria and so reaches the left heart and brain.

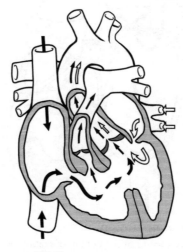

Fig. 4: Tetralogy of Fallot

Because of a blockage between the right ventricle and the pulmonary artery, some blue blood arriving in the right ventricle will cross the VSD into the left ventricle, and will reach the aorta.

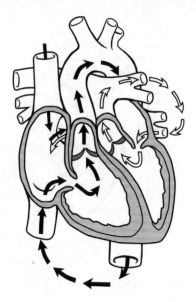

Fig. 5: Transposition of the Great Arteries (TGA)

Streaming of red and blue blood is very unfavourable: the only communication between the two sides of the heart is a hole between the atria where some blue and red blood can mix.

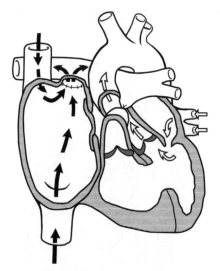

Fig. 6: A Fontan operation

This shows an early version of the Fontan operation devised to treat 'single ventricles'. The surgeon has connected the right atrium directly to the pulmonary artery and closed any hole between the atria – so blue blood arriving from the body has nowhere else to go but into the lungs. Red blood returns to the main ventricle and is pumped around the body.

ACKNOWLEDGEMENTS

Thanks to the Somerville Foundation, the American Congenital Heart Association, Little Hearts Matter, Tiny Tickers and to the Mustard and Senning Survivors Facebook group, and the various so-modern grapevines for which each serves as a hub; many patients got in touch with me having first heard about the project through these organizations. Gratitude also to several clinical colleagues who introduced me to particular people – but special thanks to Jane Somerville, Sara Thorne, Marina Hughes and Gil Wernovsky. Also to those who put me straight in other ways, especially Simon Parsons, Angus McEwan, Kate Brown, Martin Elliott, James Taylor, Gerald Graham, John Bailey, John Powell and Adelaide Tunstill.

There are others who have helped in different vital ways – encouragement, editing, nit-picking, digging through archives. Particular thanks to Jennie Condell and Penny Gardiner from Elliott and Thompson, but also to Midge Gilles, Peter Forbes, Adrian du Plessis, Becky Proctor, James Phillips and David Spiegelhalter. Thanks for your (various levels of) forbearance.

Finally and most importantly thanks to patients who have made the book what it is (the good bits that is, the failures are my own). Some will recognize their own stories, others have broadened my mind more generally.

Thanks to:
Fr Patrick Davies, Mike Shaw, Terry Shaw, Howard Holtz, Pamela
Stacherski, Sam Roeser, Sophie, Zara Majda and Nadir Ahmad,
Rajni and Ian Cairns, Charles, Janice Guise, Patrick Davies,
Xerxes Talati, Mary Jane Nichols, Marilyn Petrosie, Rita Nadeau,
Diana Sanders, Judith Parker, James Cobb, Amelia Quirke, Sian
McEwan, Gill, Michael, Olivia and Pete Smith (a.k.a 'the Smiths'),
Bernhard Reed, Christina Woodhead, Geoffrey Pollard, Guy
Mayman, Jenny Cobb, Nick Daber, James Gould, Connie Walker,
Roy Evans, Barry Butler, Richard Barnes, Susan Manley, Carol
Keyte, Steve Willoughby, Christine Rogers, Jonathan Mayman,
Kim Hammelmann and her mother, Alan Smith, Laura, Laura
Crichton, Susan Hancox, John Hunt, Chloe, Luca Allera, Liza
Morton, Gemma Searle, Sarah Clark, Paul Spencer, Tom Glenn,
Jo Murphy, Sandra Brooker, Sophie Henton, Anna Redman, Jean
Willoughby, Robert Plumridge, Wendy Knowles, Sarah Schmidt,
Simon Reuter, Samantha Goddard, Steve Graham, Louise Sharp,
Stuart Watson, Tiffiney McKee, Gail Maguire, Julie Scanes,
Paul, Suart Bonshor, Marian Brecknell, Pat Richmond, Yvonne
Seabrook, Michael Toon and several others.

REFERENCES

The sources listed below do not include references from academic medical literature.

1. Beginnings

Stoney, William, *Pioneers of Cardiac Surgery* (Nashville: Vanderbilt University Press, 2008). The full quote from Brock about Blalock's visit to Guy's Hospital (pages 7–9 in this book) can be found on page 15.

2. Minnesota, Tuesday 31 August 1954

AHC Oral History Project, University of Minnesota. In particular the work of Dominique Tobell; this includes the testimonies of Ruth Weise, R.N., M.A., Florence Marks, R.N., M.A., Theresa Sullivan, R.N., Katherine Lillehei, R.N. and John Kersey, M.D. http:/www.med.umn.edu/history/ppl/tobell/

Shaw, Terry R., *Terry Tales* (Terandlo Publishing, 2003).

Engel, Leonard, *The Operation* (London: Museum Press, 1958)

Miller, G. Wayne, *King of Hearts* (New York: Crown Publishers, 2000)

3. When nothing is done

Hoffman, Julien I. E., 'The Global Burden of Congenital Heart
Disease', *Cardiovascular Journal of Africa*, 24(4) (May 2013), 43–47

Samanek, Milan, 'Children with Congenital Heart Disease:
Probability of Natural Survival', *Pediatric Cardiology*, 13 (1992),
152–158

4. Birth was almost the death of him

UK and US antenatal diagnosis rates:

https://nicor4.nicor.org.uk/CHD/an_paeds.nsf/vwContent/
Antenatal%20Diagnosis?Opendocument

http://www.cdc.gov/ncbddd/heartdefects/features/
prenatal-diagnosis.html

5. 'Those children are my crossword puzzles'

Congenital malformations of the heart:

Taussig, Helen B., *Congenital Malformations of the Heart*, Volume 1
(Cambridge, MA: Harvard University Press, 1960)

Obituaries and reminiscences about Helen Taussig:

'Helen Brooke Taussig: 1898 to 1986', *Journal of the American College
of Cardiology*, 10(3) (September 1987), 662–71.

A piece about metallic objects flying about in MRI rooms:
http://www.simplyphysics.com/flying_objects.html

A wonderful video dealing with early fluoroscopy:
https://www.youtube.com/watch?v=CwbJS74OKes

6. When did you last see a blue baby?

Chenoweth, Alice D. and Saffian, Sadie, 'Children with Congenital
Heart Disease Served in Regional Centers, 1952–56', *Public Health
Report*, 75(5) (May 1960), 377–86.

7. Going into hospital

Bowlby J. and Robertson J., 'A Two-Year-Old Goes to Hospital',
Proceedings of the Royal Society of Medicine, 46(6) (1953), 425–427

Bakwin, Harry, 'Psychologic Aspect of Pediatrics: The Hospital Care
Of Infants And Children', *Journal of Pediatrics*, 39(3) (September
1951), 383–390

Meadow, Roy, 'The Captive Mother', *Archives of Disease in Childhood*,
44(235) (June 1969), 362

8. Magic sleep

Lorraine Sweeney as a great-grandmother remembering her operation
in 1938: https://www.youtube.com/watch?v=JOq_-L24WBs

9. Cold hearts

Warren Mauston's surgeon, Dr Samuel Hunter, quoted in Rhees, D.
and Kirk Jeffrey, 'Earl Bakken's Little White Box: The Complex
Meanings of the First Transistorized Pacemaker', via http://www.
artefactsconsortium.org/Publications/PDFfiles/Vol2Elect/2.04.
Electronics-Rhees,Jeffrey,BakkenWhiteBoxGrTotal75ppiWEBF.pdf

Ben Milstein is quoted in http://news.bbc.co.uk/1/hi/health/183660.stm

The surgeon from San Francisco is quoted in Braimbridge, M. V.,
'The International Cardiothoracic Surgeon', *Ann Thorac Surg*
(1992), 54, 193-8

The Papworth surgeon, Christopher Parish, is from the Papworth
Oral History Project, interview with Christopher Parish,
Cambridgeshire Archives Service

Pappworth, M. H., '"Human Guniea Pigs" – A History', *British
Medical Journal* 301(6766) (December 1990), 1456–60

Safar, Peter, 'Ventilatory Efficacy Of Mouth-To-Mouth Artificial
Respiration: Airway Obstruction During Manual And
Mouth-To-Mouth Artificial Respiration', *Journal of the American
Medical Association*, 167(3) (May 1958), 335–41

11. This won't hurt a bit: recovery

Reynolds L. A., and Tansey, E. M. (eds), 'History of British Intensive Care, c.1950–c.2000', *Wellcome Witnesses to Twentieth Century Medicine*, vol. 42 (London: Queen Mary, University of London, 2011)

Kelly, Fiona E; Fong, Kevin; Hirsch, Nicholas; Nolan, Jerry P., 'Intensive Care Medicine Is 60 Years Old: The History And Future Of The Intensive Care Unit', *Clinical Medicine*, 14(4) (August 2014), 376–79

Sir Gordon Gordon-Taylor quoted in Sir Thomas Holmes Sellors, 'Gordon-Taylor: His Contributions to Surgery', Lecture to the Royal College of Surgeons of England 13 June 1968, in *Annals of The Royal College of Surgeons of England*, 43(6) (January 1969), 297–312

13. Dirty washing

Gurvitz, M. et al., 'The Report of The Public Inquiry Into Children's Heart Surgery at The Bristol Royal Infirmary 1984–95: Learning From Bristol', Bristol Royal Infirmary Inquiry, 8 July 2001

14. Flying solo

'Prevalence and Predictors of Gaps in Care Among Adult Congenital Heart Disease Patients HEART-ACHD (The Health, Education, and Access Research Trial)', *Journal of the American College of Cardiology*, 61(21) (May 2013), 2180–84

'Scarred for Life', a photo exhibition of adults with congenital heart disease, mounted on behalf of the Somerville Foundation and shown in Scotland and England, (2016)

15. Grown up and trying to do normal things

Bruto, Venera C. et al., 'Determinants of Health-Related Quality of Life in Adults with Congenital Heart Disease', *Congenital Heart Disease*, 2(5) (September/October 2007), 301–13 van Rijen, E. H. M., et al., 'Psychosocial Functioning of The Adult With Congenital Heart Disease: A 20–33 Years Follow-Up', *European Heart Journal*, 24(7) (April 2003), 673–83

16. Having a baby – what's the big deal?

Oakley, Celia and Doherty, Peter, 'Pregnancy in patients after valve replacement', *British Heart Journal*, 38 (1976), 1140–48

Sanders, Diana, *Will I Still Be Me?: A Journey Through a Transplant* (Charlbury: Day Books, 2006)

17. Rhythm problems and other woes: the rise of the expert patient

http://www.philippbonhoeffer.com/first-in-man/melody-valve/

18. 'Death alone is certain, the time of death uncertain'

Goss, Rebecca, *Her Birth* (Manchester: Carcanet Press, 2013)

INDEX

A

ablation 225, 246

Adult Congenital Heart Disease
  (ACHD)
    community 5, 225, 231
    services 213–214, 253, 288

Africa 43, 99

Alder Hey scandal 263

anaesthesia/anaesthetists 3, 4, 7, 16,
    25, 115–127, 131, 137, 148,
    151, 155, 165, 167, 217
    anaesthetic explosions 121
    anaesthetic stages 122–123,
      172–173, 184–185, 264

Anderson, Patty 68

angiograms 71–72, 219

anticoagulants 202, 235–239

APGAR scores 50

arrhythmias 242–243, 246

arteries 23, 257
    arterial switch operations 277,
      279, 287, 279–280
    coronary 151–152, 154, 156,
      255, 279, 280, 281
    pulmonary (lung) 20–21,
      35–39, 54, 62, 67, 68, 92,
      120, 121, 147, 152, 179, 208,
      210, 226, 234, 252, 275, 279

see also Transposition of the
  Great Arteries

Asher, Richard 81

aspirin 238

Atrial Septal Defect (ASD) 68, 77,
    83, 133–134

Atrioventricular Septal Defect 68,
    208, 231

Attention Deficit Hyperactivity
  Disorder 91

autism 91

B

baffle operations *see* Mustard
  operations; Senning
  operations

banding 201

birth 45–56; *see also* pregnancy

Blalock, Alfred 2, 4, 7–9, 13,
    27, 30–31, 47, 65, 67, 92,
    120–122
    Blalock-Hanlon operation 277
    Blalock-Taussig shunt 66, 121

blindness, cortical 188

blood groups 14, 16, 23

blood pressure 16, 37, 38, 42, 91,
    122, 124, 267

blue children 1–3, 7–9, 12, 22,
        36–37, 47, 49, 61–64, 66,
        79–94, 176, 177, 179, 190,
        205, 209, 223, 225, 237, 266,
        277
bone marrow 23, 46
brain damage 25, 27, 112, 125,
        136, 137, 190, 191–192, 241,
        269
brain death 130, 133
breathing
    assisted 162
    rescue 131–132
    stopping 130–131
    see also ventilators
Bristol Royal Infirmary 193–194
Brock, Russell 8–9, 63, 97, 179,
        208

C
cardiac arrest 131, 188, 241, 248,
        249
Cardio-Pulmonary Resuscitation
        (CPR) 132
catheters/catheterization 12,
        69–72, 74, 225, 253
CHARGE syndrome 91
cholesterol 255, 281
circulatory arrest 137
clots/clotting 23, 25, 125, 154,
        236, 238
coarctations 54, 201, 288
congenitally corrected
        transposition 226, 234, 266,
        278–279
cosmetic surgery 7, 202, 210
Crippled Children's Hospital,
        Oklahoma 97, 120

cross-circulation 17, 22–26, 63, 79,
        126, 133, 137
cyanosis 66
cyclopropane 120–121

D
death 257–274
    brain 130, 133
    heart stopping 130, 142
    sudden cardiac 242
    see also breathing, stopping;
        resuscitation
defibrillators 118, 142, 241, 248,
        253
    Implantable Cardioverter
        Defibrillator (ICD) 225,
        242, 246, 272
    ventricular fibrillation (VF) 142
definitive palliations 204–206, 226
Dennis, Clarence 68
di George syndrome 91
dialysis 135, 268
diathermy 149–150
doping 64
    Abortion Doping 232
Down's syndrome 1, 91
Drabble, Margaret 104
drugs 23, 46, 233, 237, 242, 247,
        249, 261, 269, 284
    see also doping; named drugs
ductus operations 118–119, 125
dyslexia 91

E
Ebstein's anomaly 57–58, 180, 235,
        237, 240, 274
Edler, Inge 73–74

Eisenmenger's syndrome 40–42,
        61, 67, 234, 266–267
electrocardiogram (ECG) 15, 63,
        76, 122, 125, 131, 168, 203,
        243, 244
endocarditis 222
Enoxaparin 239
erythropoietin (EPO) 64
Extracorporeal Life Support (ECLS)
        144–145
Extracorporeal Membrane
        Oxygenation (ECMO) 145

F
Facebook 34, 94, 256, 259, 271,
        283
    Mustard and Senning Survivors
    Group 282–287, 290
Fallot's tetralogy 5, 13 17, 18, 20,
        22, 29–30, 32, 43, 65, 66,
        77, 79, 99, 141, 147–157,
        176, 179, 209, 210, 221, 223,
        244, 245, 248, 253, 288, *295*
fetal heart 47–51, 54–55, 202,
        295
fluoroscopy 64
Fontan operations 205, 207, 208,
        219, 223, 226, 227, 244,
        271–272, *296*
Forssmann, Werner 69
Franklin D. Roosevelt School for
        Physically Disabled Children
        90
Freud, Anna 101

G
Gibbon, Dr 68

Glenn, Dr 208
Gordon-Taylor, Sir Gordon 171
Goss, Rebecca 273
Great Ormond Street Hospital 71,
        104, 109, 135
Gross, Dr 119
Grown-Up Congenital Heart
        Disease (GUCH) *see* Adult
        Congenital Heart Disease
        (ACHD)
Guy's Hospital 8, 57, 68, 97

H
haemoglobin 36
Hammersmith Hospital 99, 139
Harriet Lane Home for Invalid
        Children 62
Harvard Medical School 69
heart
    block 143
    failure 254, 279
    murmurs 39, 62, 254
    rhythms 207, 241–256, 271,
        272–273, 281
    see also arrhythmias
heart-lung machines 26, 27, 133,
        138, 139, 142, 150, 151
heparin 150, 236
Hertz, Helmuth 73–74
Holtz, Howard 14, 16–18, 21–22,
        26
hospitals 95–113, 132, 159, 162,
        166, 172, 181, 192, 199,
        210–212, 235, 236, 238,
        248, 259, 263, 269, 282, 288,
        289
    see also named hospitals
hypertension *see* blood pressure

Hypoplastic Left Heart Syndrome
       (HLHS) 5, 32, 54, 77,
       171–172, 183–184, 207,
       219–220, 262–265
hypothermia 135–137

I

Implantable Cardioverter Defibrillator
       (ICD) 225, 242, 246
India 34, 99
intensive care units (ICU)
       160–164, 166–175, 184–186,
       241, 258, 268–269
iron lung 164
Italy 24

J

Jefferson Medical College 138
Johns Hopkins Hospital 2, 7, 57,
       62, 66, 131, 135
Johns Hopkins Medical School 61,
       23

K

keloids 202
Kennedy, Patrick Bouvier 163, 167
Ket, Dick 29–32, 43, 66, 79
keyhole surgery 201
kidney(s) 64, 135, 239–240, 268
    failure 23, 24, 135
    see also dialysis
knots 156–157

L

Lank, Betty 119

leukaemia 23–24
Lillehei, Dr 16, 21–22, 65, 134,
       143, 153
Liston, Robert 25

M

Madhubala 32–34, 38–40, 42, 43, 67
Magnetic Resonance Imaging
       (MRI) 75–76
Maids Morton Convalescent Home
       179
Mauston, Warren 129
McLeod, Hugh 276
Middlesex Hospital 171
Milstein, Ben 134
morbus caeruleus 62
Mustard operations 144, 163, 244,
       276–286, 288

N

National Health Service (NHS)
       97–98, 193, 266
Nazis 135, 262
Norwood, Dr 262
    operations 207, 219

O

organ donation 263
    see also Alder Hey scandal
oxygen tents 166
oxygenators 138, 139–140, 144

P

pacemakers 129, 143, 144, 203,
       225, 237, 245–247, 287

palpitations 57–58, 242
  see also arrhythmias
Papworth Hospital 134, 139–140
Pargetter, Elizabeth 83
Percutaneous Pulmonary Valve
    Implantation (PPVI) 225,
    252–253
pneumothorax 169
polio 15, 89, 161, 164
  see also iron lung
Post Traumatic Stress Disorder
    175
potassium solution 142, 152
pregnancy 24, 34, 42, 49, 51,
    52, 84, 137, 209, 223, 228,
    231–240, 261, 265, 276,
    284
  termination 265
prostaglandins 55–56
pulmonary atresia 5, 32, 54, 55,
    176, 211
pulmonary stenosis 54, 83,
    253–254

R
Rashkind, Bill 53
Rastelli operations 204
recovery 159–177
resuscitation 46, 132–133, 142,
    215, 238, 241, 249, 259
  Cardio-Pulmonary
    Resuscitation (CPR)
    132
  'Do not resuscitate' order
    (DNR) 259
Robertson, James 101–102
Royal College of Surgeons 7, 8,
    171

S
Saxon, Eileen 9
Sellors, Thomas Holmes 171
Senning operations 163, 223, 228,
    244, 247, 278, 280–284, 286,
    287
septum
  atrial 208, 231
  ventricular 208, 215, 231
Shaw, Mickey 12–22, 26, 27, 30,
    47, 79, 126, 134, 137, 153,
    201
Shore, David 136
shunt(s) 38, 40, 55, 65, 66, 68,
    163, 176, 190, 203, 223
  Blalock-Taussig 66, 121
  operations 27, 31, 62, 92, 97,
    120, 225
Somerville, Jane 213–214
special schools 89, 188
stem-cell grafts 291
sternotomy 202, 203
stitching/stitches 7, 153, 179, 244,
    281
strokes 42, 258
support groups 289–291
  see also Facebook, Mustard and
    Senning Survivors Group

T
Taussig, Helen 7, 61–62, 64–67,
    69, 76, 213, 262
  Blalock-Taussig shunt 66, 121
Tavistock Clinic 101
teratogens 237
tetralogy of Fallot *see* Fallot's tetralogy
thalidomide 237
Thomas, Vivien 66

Total Anomalous Pulmonary
    Venous Drainage/
    Connection (TAPVD/C)
    32, 47, 54
Total Cavo Pulmonary Connection
    205, 272
tracheostomy 164–167
transplants 145, 204, 263, 267,
    271–272, 284, 286, 287, 290
    see also Alder Hey scandal
Transposition of the Great Arteries
    (TGA) 32, 52, 54, 67, 144,
    163, 229, 241, 244, 247, 275,
    277–281, 281, 284, 286, 290,
    296
    congenitally corrected
    transposition 234, 266,
    278–279
Truman, Harry S. 20
Truncus Arteriosus 204, 205
2D echo machines 72–76, 155

U
ultrasound scans 49, 51, 52, 55, 56,
    73–75, 84, 239, 265
University of Minnesota Heart
    Hospital 15, 20

V
valves 36, 47, 62, 99, 210, 225, 234,
    236, 238, 251, 252, 253, 291

aortic 76, 136, 209
mitral 209
Percutaneous Pulmonary Valve
    Implantation (PPVI) 225,
    252–253
pulmonary 38, 136, 154, 179,
    190, 200, 210, 225, 250–251,
    253–254
tricuspid 57, 72, 152, 154, 237,
    239, 279, 281
Varco, Dr 16
ventilators 167–168, 215, 241, 259,
    268, 269, 278
ventricular
    Assist Device (VAD) 145
    fibrillation (VF) 142
    Septal Defect (VSD) 5, 32–34,
    38–41, 43, 67, 92, 143, 147,
    152, 154, 163, 200, 232,
    266, *294*

W
Wambo, Arnaud 43
warfarin 236–238
Watson, Stuart 286
Westminster Hospital 136
Wood, Paul 131

X
X-rays 15, 64, 69–71, 201, 247,
    252, 277